Darla
Faith Over Fire

by

Darla, Roger and Mardell Hansen

as told to

Bev Larsen

Heritage Publishers, Inc.
Flagstaff, Arizona

For additional copies of this book please contact:

Roger Hansen   or   Darla Hansen
Rt. 1   Rt. 1, Box 71
Brayton, IA 50042   Elk Horn, IA 51531
(712) 549-2345

Darla, Faith Over Fire

Copyright © 1991 Darla Hansen
Heritage Publishers, Inc.
2700 Woodlands Village Boulevard, Suite 300
Flagstaff, Arizona 86001-7124
(602) 526-1129

All rights reserved. No part of this publication may be reproduced or transmitted in any form or by any means, electronic or mechanical, including photocopying, recording, or by any information storage and retrieval system, without permission in writing from Darla Hansen and Heritage Publishers, Inc.

ISBN 0-929690-13-3
Library of Congress Cataloging Number 91-76295

Printed and bound in the United States of America

Contents

IF ONLY	1
ENTERING THE VALLEY	6
THE SHADOW OF DEATH	12
ON TO TEXAS	20
DAY BY DAY	31
PREJUDICE	42
ANOTHER LOSS	44
KAPTAIN KWIK	46
GOODBYE TEXAS	48
HOME AGAIN	53
ADJUSTMENTS	56
MOVING ON	75
PHASE TWO	79
SCHOOL YEARS	83
THE SOUND OF MUSIC	86
LESSONS	88
MOVING—WITH RESERVATIONS	95
DEREK	99
CHANGE OF PLANS	103
WEDDING BELLS	105
SETTLING IN	108
MOTHERHOOD	113
MUSIC, MUSIC	116
CHOICES	119
ON THE MOUNTAIN TOP	122

Dedications

To my mother, Christina Hoegh, who moved into our home those four and a half months and cared for our older children. I have thanked you many times, Mom, but "Thanks again!"

And, to my husband, Roger, you had the most difficult task of trying to be in two places at once, at home in Iowa with our older children and in Texas with Darla and me. You always seemed to know where you were needed most.

Mardell

To our other children, July, Ken, Connie, Jeff and Lori. We kind of deserted you those four and a half months but you all adjusted well. We know you were neglected at times and we are sorry. You know we would have done the same had it been any of you. You have made us very proud parents and we love you.

To our daughter, Darla, what a brave little four year old you were! Hardly a whimper, and always a "Thank you." When we asked, "How are you?" the answer was always "Fine." We didn't take care of you, Darla, you took care of us! What a joy you are. We love you.

Mom and Dad

I would like to dedicate this book to the loving memory of Edward "Ted" Cutler, Potentate of the Des Moines ZA-GA-ZIG Shriners the year I was burned. He was much more than that to me, though. Through the years he became "Grandpa Ted" to me. Because of his wisdom and love I learned much and became a better person. I miss you, Ted.

I would also like to pay a gigantic "Thank you" to my parents, Roger and Mardell. No words can describe the love and respect that I have for you both. I cannot fathom how you could go through all that you did with my illness. The initial four and a half months of totally uprooting your lives for me and the 14 following years of treatment that you sacrificed to help me through. God really knew what he was doing when he chose you to be my parents. I love you very much!

Darla

To the Shriners of North America and especially the ZA-GA-ZIG Temple of Des Moines, Iowa, your generosity to burned and crippled children is immeasurable. Your care and concern for Darla and our entire family during these years is most appreciated!

Mardell, Roger and Darla

Foreword

It has been close to one year since *Faith Over Fire* was first published. I have had so many exciting experiences since then that I wanted to update you. . . so perhaps it would be more appropriate to call this a "Backward" rather than a Foreword.

The debut of the book took place on November 4, 1990. This was the 24th anniversary of my accident. I had been wanting to do a gospel concert at my church, Elk Horn Lutheran Church, Elk Horn, Iowa, and this seemed the perfect time. About one week before the concert we put up a few posters around town and an announcement appeared in three area newspapers. The night before, we set up fifty chairs in the church thinking that there would be several empty ones. Well, was I surprised and overwhelmed when there were well over 300 people in attendance! I wanted to do something special for my parents so I wrote them a song called "Thank You for the Love." It was one of the easiest songs I've ever written, but one of the hardest to sing. It was a very emotional, but wonderful day.

After that day, groups began asking me to speak and sing. I have met so many people and traveled to many places. Some of the most memorable include several Shriners' events, including speaking to the football players at the Iowa Shrine High School Football Banquet and singing the National Anthem at the football game in the Unidome in Cedar Falls, Iowa. I have spoken to many students including the West Interstate 80 Junior High Leadership Academy and a Future Homemakers of America Camp. I feel especially fortunate to be able to tell these young people that they don't have to be just like everyone else; to be comfortable with who they are; and not to be ashamed of their faith.

In April 1991 the Shriners' Burn Institute in Galveston, Texas had a 25-year reunion. My parents and I were able to attend this two-day event. Over 2,000 patients, employees, and Shriners were there. It was so wonderful to see my plastic surgeon, Dr. Duane Larson, Sara Bolieu of the Institute's public relations department, and so many of my former nurses and fellow patients. I was impressed by the fact that so many of the employees who worked there when I was a patient are still there. The nurse who cared for me on the first night I arrived is still working there. She clearly remembered the night and told me that I didn't complain, but kept on saying, "You don't do things like they do back home."

There is a new Shriners' Burn Unit being built only a few blocks from the old one. It is bigger, with more modern equipment to help save many more burn victims. It is scheduled to open in 1992.

I am a fitness instructor because I believe that exercise is a very important aspect of life. I strive to educate others on the benefits it can bring to their lives. In May 1991 I was honored as the recipient of the IDEA Christine MacIntyre Memorial Award. Christine MacIntyre was the founding editor of *Shape* Magazine. The award is given annually to a fitness professional who has overcome a handicap or hardship to achieve and promote high standards in fitness. My friend and co-worker, Denise Reinig, wrote a letter to the association for fitness nominating me. After reviewing over 200 nominations IDEA narrowed the field to twelve including me. They interviewed me by phone from San Diego asking my views on fitness and life. One week later, I was notified that they had chosen me. I was presented the award at a ceremony at IDEA'a International Conference in Nashville on May 31, 1991. I was given an engraved plaque and a donation of $1,000 was given in my name to the charity of my choice. I chose the Shriners' Burn Hospital in Galveston.

In my acceptance speech I stressed that exercise and fitness are vital for good health, not just for losing weight and looking good. Not everyone can look perfect, but we must be the best we can be. As fitness professionals we must help others to understand and accept this concept. Joe Weider wrote an article about me in *Shape*'s December 1991 issue.

"Girls Nite Out," Nancy and I, are still singing performing at everything from rodeos to dances to high school fund-raisers. We finished in the top eight out of 74 acts in Omaha's WOW Country Music Showdown.

Derek and I celebrated our ten-year wedding anniversary this year. Our children, Monica is in the first grade and Jordan is in pre-school. My parents and siblings remain close and enjoy time together often.

As you can see, it has been a wonderful year! I do truly feel blessed by God for what he has done for me and continues to do.

God Bless You!
Darla

CHAPTER 1

IF ONLY....

An autumn haze hung over western Iowa that early morning of November 4, 1966. In a very few days, a shifting weather pattern would bring sleet and frozen rain, icing over roads and making driving hazardous.

This Friday, though, still clung to the last vestige of Indian summer. Gray, cloudy and still, the sky hinted at the change to come, with intermittent bursts of sun through the dismal sky.

In Audubon County, half way between Des Moines, the state capital, and Omaha, Nebraska, corn picking was well under way and the yield was good. The weather had cooperated, with no frustrating days of mud which had slowed harvest the past several years.

It was 7:15 a.m., and rural mothers were calling hurry-up messages to children who would soon need to meet school buses at the end of country lanes.

Roger Hansen, a farmer in southern Oakfield Township, had gotten up before sunrise, grumbling a bit to himself about Daylight Savings Time. He had now finished his hog chores, attended to a few minor adjustments on the corn picker, and eaten the good breakfast his wife, Mardell, had prepared.

Of their large family, only the oldest and youngest would not be riding the school bus that day. Judy, 19, who would later graduate at the top of her class, was in training at Jennie Edmundson School of Nursing in Council Bluffs, 50 miles to the west. Darla, the baby of the six, had just turned four years old on Monday, October 31.

Seventeen year old Ken was a senior at Elk Horn-Kimballton Community School. Connie, at 13, was an eighth grader; Jeff, nine, was a fourth grader, and Lori, seven, who for several years had been "the baby", was now in second grade.

Happy that it was Friday, the four gathered up assorted notebooks, musical instruments, "show and tell" items, and their lunch boxes.

Darla, still in her nightgown, wistfully watched them go, from her perch, kneeling on a chair pushed up to the window. She was lonesome for Judy, and as her four other siblings left for school each day, she wished with all her little heart that it could be summer all the time, when she would not be the only one at home. Or that she were old enough to climb on the big yellow bus with the others. The four outside, hearing the familiar grind of the bus, turned and waved at her one last time.

As he got up from the table, Roger glanced out the window over Darla's head and noticed a flat tire on the corn wagon. It would have to be fixed immediately. Until it was, picking would be at a standstill.

He hurried outside, jacked up the empty wagon, removed the tire and got it into the box of his pickup truck.

"Anything you need in town?" he hollered to his wife.

"No!" she answered from the porch steps. She was aware of how stressful are harvest delays. "Anything I should do here? Do you want me to throw hay to the cattle?!"

"Sure would help," he answered. He glanced at the sky, hoping the weather would hold a few more days. Then he was off to town, not too far behind the school bus.

Inside, Mardell was pulling on her chore boots. "Can you be a good girl and play with your toys 'till Mama comes back in?"

Still sleepy, Darla nodded her promise. Mardell had the fleeting thought that her youngest no doubt would get a blanket off her bed and curl up on the sofa with her favorite doll and watch Captain Kangaroo. It was too cold to bring her along outside without taking the time to completely dress her. Besides, like thousands of other farm children all over the country, she had often stayed in the house alone.

The porch door slammed. Bored, the little girl sat now at the kitchen table, swinging her bare feet and legs, daydreaming of what to do. She rested her blond head on her arms, thinking of her birthday party the previous Sunday. The day-early celebration had filled the farmhouse with grandparents, aunts, uncles and cousins. She remembered the fun, the presents, the food. . . . .

Gum. That's what she wanted now. She hopped down and looked about her for her mother's purse. She knew her mother had just bought some Fruit Stripe gum and it was her favorite. She spied the purse on top of the refrigerator.

She dragged a kitchen chair from the table and pushed it against the refrigerator. Standing on tiptoe and stretching so- hard, she finally touched the handle and pulled it down.

Darla settled down with it on the couch. The brass snap was tight and her tiny fingers could not possibly make it budge. She sighed. What to do now? Ah, here along the side was something she had overlooked before. Interesting. A nice long zipper. How she loved working zippers! She sat for a time, moving it back and forth, enjoying the feel of the movement, postponing any look inside.

But at last she tired of zipping, and peered into the pocket. Hmm...her fingers felt about for gum. Nothing at all promising here. And then, stuck in one corner, a small packet of matches.

Mardell and Roger had dined out one evening with their card club before corn picking had started and picked them up at a cafe in Winterset. Neither of them smoked, but the matches were attractive, done in black and metallic gold. The colors complimented the name of the establishment which included the word "gold".

"Pretty souvenir," Mardell had remarked as she slipped them into her purse, "even if we won't ever use them."

And oh, they were pretty. The prettiest matches Darla had ever seen. Not at all like the plain ones your buy at the grocery store. These tips were golden, with sparkly stuff like a fairy would have on her wand. . . .

Maybe, just maybe, if Darla could make this first match make a fire, it would sparkle so brightly that a fairy would come to see it, and dance around the room with her wand making shiny sparks to match. Maybe the fairy would talk to her, and stay to play. . . .

With effort, she removed the first one. She held the rest in her other hand and scraped the golden tip against the black rectangle.

At once, the tip ignited. She watched it, fascinated. But so quickly the match burned down. Down to her little finger tips. She felt the first awful pain and tried to blow it out. Being frightened, she instinctively dropped it, as well as the rest of the matches, onto her lap. A lap of flannel nightgown material stretched across her legs.

Immediately, she was engulfed in a wicked blaze, which in seconds destroyed nightgown, underpants, and most of her skin, with the exception of the soles of her feet, below her knees and her face.

Her pitiful screams echoed through the empty house.

CHAPTER 2
ENTERING THE VALLEY

With nothing more to feed upon, the flames burned themselves out. Darla, driven by some primitive instinct, had fled to the bathroom, seeking water. Once there, the fire was over. And her reach was too short to work the faucets without climbing into the tub.

In shock, she somehow made her way to the porch, knowing her mother would soon be back. And in a few minutes she was, coming up the walk and seeing her youngest dimly through the glass in the door. As she drew closer she could see no nightgown.

"She looked," Mardell says today, "as though she had on a pair of old leotards from the play clothes box we kept upstairs. That was my first thought, because, aside from her face, she was <u>dark brown</u>. . . . ."

As she stepped up into the porch, there was the faint smell of burning, and as she looked closely, she realized the silent four-year-old child had been horribly, cruelly burned.

Mardell was afraid to touch her, somehow knowing that the slightest pressure would make the skin fall off of her. Trying to hide her fear from the child, Mardell guided her back into the house. She grabbed a clean Elk Horn-Kimballton sweatshirt of Judy's, which was hanging over the back of a chair and gently dropped it over Darla's head. It hung on the little body like a gunny sack.

She dialed the number of Earl Madsen's DX station with shaky hands, fighting off her own light-headedness. She knew it was up to her to do what must be done until she could find Roger and medical help.

She fought back hysteria and said into the phone, "Don't let Roger Hansen leave there! Darla's been hurt and we have to go to the hospital!"

Over and over she told herself: I've got to stay calm for Darla. Help me, Lord, to be calm, and to drive. Mother and daughter walked to the car, Darla not saying a word. Mardell drove at normal speed into town, six miles north. She knew if she drove faster than normal she might have an accident, and there would be delay in getting help.

Roger was waiting at the curb. The tire, the truck were forgotten now. He took the driver's seat, and drove quickly to the home of Dr. Gerald Larson, just three blocks from the station.

But the doctor had gone before dawn to Myrtue Memorial Hospital at Harlan, some 15 miles away. Mrs. Larson told them: "Start for the hospital and I'll call and have them keep him there until you come."

Suddenly, Mardell remembered her fear that there might be something on fire at the house--perhaps the whole house might be in flames! She flung open the car door and called to Mrs. Larson, "Our house may be on fire -- I'm not sure -- call the neighbors!"

Jeanette Larson tried each one of the Hansen's closest neighbors, without luck. No one answered. Each household's phone rang and rang, as the occupants were outside, busy at morning chores, or at harvesting in the field.

Jeanette and son, Bob, who had not yet left for school, hurried into their car and drove swiftly to the Hansen farm.

They found no actual fire, but the crocheted rug on which Darla had sat was smoldering. Jeanette scooped it up and put it to soak in the tub. They made a quick check of the rest of the house to see there were no other problems, no iron left on, or stove burner.

Meanwhile, as the Hansens left Elk Horn, Roger realized that the car was low on gas. He therefore swung into the station at Kimballton, the other Danish village, just three miles north of Elk Horn.

Alvin Johnson, the owner of the station could see that the child, sitting between her parents had a medical emergency. He moved quickly to fill the tank. "Go!" he ordered Roger, when the latter fumbled for his billfold. "Just go -- pay me some other time!" Roger says when he went back some months later to pay him, Alvin said, "You don't have a bill here!"

They sped toward the hospital, heading west on Highway 44. Only a few miles out of town, they recognized the car coming toward them from the opposite direction was the familiar Volkswagon, which was the doctor's trademark. He had apparently left the hospital before the message could be delivered.

Roger wheeled the car around, heading back east, following the doctor, honking the horn, with Mardell frantically waving her arm out the window.

At last, Dr. Larson spied them in his rear-view mirror. He slowed, both cars reversed direction and sped toward the hospital. At this point the doctor did not know the particulars, only that something was terribly wrong.

During all of this, Darla was not in pain. In shock, she sat silently between her parents, waiting, quiet, far-away.

Lois Wirth was on duty in admitting that morning. She glanced up from the chart she was checking as Dr. Larson, who had just passed her desk a few minutes before, heading for Elk Horn, re-entered the hospital, at a slow run, carrying a small child in his arms.

Within minutes, emergency room examination revealed that the child would require more sophisticated care than this small rural hospital could provide. Darla was therefore sent by ambulance to Children's Hospital in Omaha, with the doctor at her side, and the parents following in their car.

Darla's only comment to Dr. Larson was "My butt hurts..." Her feeling there had not been completely destroyed because the damage on that part of her body was "only" second degree burns.

That year, the long awaited Interstate 80 was very slowly pushing its way across western Iowa. South and east of the Hansen farm was the westernmost point of pavement. Giant machines -- bulldozers, dumptrucks and dirt scrapers were working this November day.

Had the Interstate been finished through Iowa, the trip to Omaha would have taken much less time. As it was, the ambulance followed State Highway #83 through Avoca, Hancock and other villages, on through Council Bluffs, before crossing the Missouri River bridge which led into Omaha.

By the time the two vehicles reached the city, it was mid-morning and the rush hour traffic had luckily thinned. It was still moderate to heavy at certain intersections. A series of stoplights served to slow the flow. The ambulance driver elected not to put on the flashing red light. According to the doctor, Darla was not at that hour in a life-threatening condition. Her prognosis was very poor, obviously. But she was not in immediate danger of dying before they reached the hospital.

At Children's Hospital, the doctors were blunt. "Your child is very severely burned. There is no hope that she will survive. She will no doubt get through today, and perhaps through the night. But be prepared that she will go tomorrow."

To have the doctors put it into so many words made it a terrifying reality. This was the way it was going to be. They would lose their baby. Within hours, their youngest would be torn from them.

Darla was wheeled into one of three isolation rooms. Mardell and Roger were given sterile gowns. Before putting his on, Roger made a series of calls to family members and to neighbors, asking someone to call Rev. Eugene Wekander, their pastor at the Elk Horn Lutheran Church.

He then joined Mardell at their daughter's bedside. They had no idea then just what a long, long vigil it would be.

Unable to touch her, they clung to each other. "How long?" they each asked themselves silently. "How many more hours will Darla be alive?"

CHAPTER 3
THE SHADOW OF DEATH

Just a few miles to the east, Judy was busy doing clinical work as a student nurse at Jennie Edmundson Memorial Hospital. A supervisor interrupted her concentration. "There's a call for you, Schrader," she announced and bustled on her way.

Judy went cold with apprehension. Her husband, Jerry, was in the Air Force at Monterey, California, taking an intense Chinese language program. Was something wrong? Was he being sent overseas?

Nursing students were not allowed to receive phone calls. If this call got through, something was terribly wrong.

Then -- her father's voice. Mother! It was always Mother that called!

"No, it's not Mom," Roger said. "It's Darla." His voice came over the line, choking with emotion. "She's badly burned and she's here at Childrens' Hospital..."

"I'm coming right away!"

A classmate offered to drive her, but Judy wanted her own transportation. In a daze, she was soon bucking the noon traffic, heading across the bridge to Omaha.

And then there were three to sit at Darla's bedside. To sit and to pray and to speak words of comfort to the little child, drifting in and out of consciousness, and looking so very small in the big bed.

For the first 36 hours, she was conscious, speaking in a soft voice to her mother, father, or Judy, curious about what was happening to her and often asking about the siblings at home. Sometimes the one at the bedside and Darla joined in a wavering duet of "Jesus Loves Me."

And then the dreaded turn. She slipped, silently, gently, into a coma. The exhausted family members prayed and wept, stared out the hospital windows, walked as through a bad dream up and down the hall, returning to resume the vigil.

Her eyes were now swollen shut. The horrible thought that this is how she might look very soon, lying in a small white coffin, came to all three of them -- a thought so awful that none shared it with the others until much later.

The weary, battered little body needed more than mere sleep. It could only find its rejuvenating rest by going deep into the mysterious, intangible place where no human voice can reach, no stimulus can force a reaction.

Then, midway through the second day of the coma, speaking no louder than at any other time, saying nothing other than she had said countless times before, Mardell murmured to her, "Darla, you need to get well, 'cause you're my best friend!"

Somehow the message of maternal love broke through the mist. Slowly the child struggled back to consciousness. Weakly but clearly the words came: "But, Mommy, Jesus is our very best friend. That's what the teacher said in Sunday School." Exhausted from that faint effort, Darla fell into a normal sleep.

Mardell and Roger, in their sterile gowns, hugged each other. "She'll make it now!" Roger's voice was husky with unshed tears.

Darla's head had now swollen to the size of a basketball. Her parents feared that this was an indication of brain damage. Or were her injuries so severe and her time so short, that it didn't matter, anyway? Perhaps all that was pertinent was "How long does she have left?"

In that time, could they somehow convey to her that they all loved her so much, and that Jesus Himself would be waiting to receive her into her new heavenly home?

Judy was able to work out a way to make Darla more comfortable, if only a tiny measure. She seemed to respond, with minute indications that only a family member would recognize, when this way of changing the wrappings was less stressful than another. The night nurses seemed happy for her suggestions.

But in the morning, an instructor came in with several student nurses to change the "soaks". Judy, standing nearby, leaned over her sister's tiny frame and made a suggestion as to what seemed to work best. The instructor crooked an eyebrow and replied, "Thanks anyway, but we'll follow the usual procedure."

The sarcasm was very noticeable. But no matter, Judy thought, Darla had survived the first night and at that moment nothing else really mattered.

Dr. McLaughlin was in charge of the treatment. His patient was wrapped in gauze and soaked repeatedly with a solution of silver nitrate, the same fluid that is dropped into the eyes of newborns. Blood and plasma was injected into her, and together with the monitoring devices, formed a tangle of tubes leading from her body to the carts at either side of the bed.

On Sunday afternoon, the four siblings had come to see her. Barred from her room, as a precaution against infection, they stood at the large window of her room and peered sadly in at their little sister. Mardell stood to the side, weeping, feeling that this might very well be the last time Ken, Jeff, Lori and Connie would see her alive.

For despite her prayers that her child be spared, Mardell felt in her heart that they would lose Darla. The doctors were so very pessimistic, and she had no reason not to face reality based on what they said. Roger, however, had never believed that she would not somehow miraculously pull through these terrible days and live.

On Monday morning Roger sat, half-dozing in a big chair by the bed. One of the doctors came in, with a knife, and without a word, bent over Darla and began making slits on her narrow, discolored chest.

This was a procedure necessary for relieving the pressure from fluids which were constantly building up under the burned shell. Standing now, on the other side of the bed, the father watched, agonizing over the pain his youngest was enduring, wishing fervently he could have undergone this for her.

The young doctor, looking at him across the bed gave Roger a grin. "There's more than one way to skin a cat!"

The look on Roger's face -- of shock and disgust -- revealed to the other man how thoughtless he must have sounded. Roger continued to stare at him a moment and then strode out of the room.

He leaned heavily against the wall just outside the door and thought: She's at their mercy. . . .I mustn't. . . .I can't say anything!. . . .He didn't mean anything. . . .Just bad judgement. . . .She can't make it without them. . . .and she will make it. . . .God is merciful. . .She's in His hands.

When the young man at last left the room, he glanced at Roger. Roger gave him a cool nod, that he hoped would pass for a civil one. He took his place beside Darla once again and hoped Mardell was getting a nap as she took her break in the lobby.

* * * * * * * * * * * *

Winter was whirling down on Iowa and Nebraska. Temperatures plummeted, though the snowfall, in keeping with the cycle of dryness the area was undergoing, was less than normal.

Loyal friends and family members took turns driving to Omaha to show their support. They brought fresh clothing, took verbal and written instructions back to Elk Horn, and found what errands could be done to spare Grandmother Hoegh and the children. Mardell's mother, Christena Hoegh had taken it upon herself to move in at the farm when the accident happened. Widowed in 1961 when her husband, Eddy, died, she knew that she was needed to help with the children remaining at home. Roger's parents, George and Louise Hansen, were living in Atlantic and already elderly, so were not as able to pitch in.

Mardell's brother and sister-in-law, Calvin and Phyllis Hoegh, stopped on their way to the hospital and bought two new dresses for Mardell, knowing she had left home with nothing besides what she had been wearing for chores, old blue jeans and a plaid shirt.

Another brother, Emery Hoegh, was asked to find Darla's life insurance premium notice, due on her birthday. He found the notice and took care of the premium. Making out checks and balancing the check book were the last things Mardell and Roger could handle then.

Pastor Eugene Wekander of the Elk Horn Lutheran Church and Pastor Clayton Nielsen of Omaha were of indispensable spiritual help to Roger and Mardell.

Their visits, prayers, and counsel, their willingness to just listen through the fears and uncertainties, became sources of strength and reinforcement to their faith.

Sometimes, alone and distraught, Mardell would go into the hospital chapel and find solace at the organ, playing familiar hymns and quietly singing or just silently reminding herself of the words of comfort found in the verses.

For the first five nights of Darla's time in Omaha, when her life was hanging by a very slender thread, Roger and Mardell remained in the hospital, using one of the isolation rooms, which adjoined hers. On the sixth day, to clear the room for possible emergency need, they had to move to a rooming house three blocks from the hospital.

One evening, a cousin, Darlene Schrader and her husband Harley insisted the Hansens drive to their Omaha home for supper. It took much convincing for both of them felt guilty for leaving Darla, but Judy would be at her bedside, and Dr. McLaughlin, hearing about the invitation, came in with a mock stern manner and ordered them to go.

Back home, the Hansen farm chores and harvest went on smoothly, thanks to neighbors, friends and relatives. There was a rallying around, as occurs only in rural America. Hogs, cattle and chickens were taken care of, feed was ground, and manure scooped, according to a schedule that was set up by those responsible for helping.

The last of the crop was harvested. Wives of the workers prepared and served gigantic meals and mid-morning and afternoon coffee-break pastries. Some of these volunteers themselves had been recipients of similar help when health or other family emergencies upset farm routine. Now it was their turn to reciprocate. Roger and Mardell had often pitched in where needed. They had seen their parents respond to such needs, and it was for them, as for those who were now helping them, a thing taken for granted. It was part of their way of life in rural Iowa.

A fund was started at the Shelby County State Bank in Elk Horn and another at the Elk Horn Lutheran Church to help defray expenses.

Then, without announcing their intentions, two Shriners came to the Hansens on an errand of mercy. They told them of the brand new Burn Center at Galveston where children such as Darla are cared for at no cost to the family.

Techniques had been refined there over the years, due to the many experiences the staff had with victims horribly burned in oil field explosions.

The Omaha doctors knew this was the best thing to do and encouraged the move as they tried to strengthen Darla for the trip.

The doctors there would later highly praise their fellow practitioners at Omaha who had brought Darla through the first 15 days. They then assumed the burden of rebuilding 85% of Darla's body.

CHAPTER 4
ON TO TEXAS

TV Station KMTV was on hand with reporter and cameraman to record for the viewers this turning point in the fragile life of the little girl whose latest development was being covered on radio, TV and newspapers.

The small aircraft pulled up and away from Eppley Airfield in Omaha, climbing west into the headwind before veering south. On the ground Roger and Shriners Ted Cutler, Charlie Pope, and Howard Juel waved goodbye.

Aboard, besides the pilot and the patient, were Mardell and two registered nurses. Unknown to Mardell and Roger was the expectation by the Omaha doctors that Darla would not survive the trip. Yet they had insisted that she make the trip, feeling that her chances were enhanced by her doing so.

The flight was uneventful until they were almost at their destination. Fog hung low over south Texas as they flew closer to the Gulf of Mexico. The three women suspended conversation in order to hear the pilot and the controller at the tower exchange ideas on the possibility of turning back to Houston, some 50 miles inland.

Mardell felt tenseness through her back and shoulders. "Is it going to be too foggy to land in Galveston?"

Straining his eyes ahead, the pilot called to her over his shoulder, "I think we can make it!"

Almost in unison the three women chorused: "Don't press your luck!" They smiled at each other over their identical reactions.

On the tarmac, an ambulance waited for Darla, and she was sped away within minutes. A hospital employee took Mardell to a rooming house some four blocks from the hospital.

The moment they drove up in front of it, Mardell was filled with uneasiness. Huge untrimmed bushes flanked the walkway. She could just imagine someone jumping out at her when she came back after dark, tired from a day spent at the hospital. Well, it would have to do for now. Leaving her suitcase in the middle of the room, she hurried to Darla.

The examination and consultation lasted several hours. Afterwards, Mardell was told there was only a five percent chance that Darla would survive. That seemed more promising than to say that there was a 95% chance that she would die.

Finding a pay phone, she called Roger. Between sobs, she explained the dismal prognosis.

"I'll be there some time tomorrow," he promised.

Darla had been placed in a private room, on a bed with a built-in scale, so that she could be weighed without being moved. A half-moon shaped "cradle" was over the bed, made of curved folding steel. Draped over the cradle, the bedcovers were arranged so that Darla was kept warm, but there could be no irritation, and subsequent infection to the burns.

She was cold much of the time, and a heat lamp was put under the tent for additional warmth.

Fighting the pain, she constantly ground her teeth together, so that her two bottom baby teeth in the front loosened and came out prematurely.

Seeing her mother she whispered, "We had the sirens on, Mama," and then, "Did you see the palm trees?" Mardell was surprised that she knew what palm trees were, let alone that she was alert enough to see them out the ambulance windows.

Mardell bedded down on a chair-bed the staff brought in. She fell asleep counting the hours until Roger would walk through the door. She did not want to return to the boarding house alone.

After the first few nights, parents were not allowed to remain in the hospital overnight. The Hansens were to find that this regulation was a wise one. It forced the parents to get out and away from the stress. To get back to their rooms, to a cafe, fresh air, and rest. If they remained at the hospital around the clock each day their own health and sanity would be at risk.

Early the following morning Mardell went into the hospital cafeteria for coffee. A young couple seated at the next table spotted her at once as a parent new to the hospital routine.

"Come over and join us," the woman invited.

Gratefully, Mardell brought her tray over and the Kohlers from North Dakota introduced themselves. Their son, Todd, seven, was receiving treatment for burns on his chest and arm.

When Mardell voiced her wish to be in a better rooming house, her new friends went into action.

"You're going to come where we are!" Jeanie Kohler declared. "There's several empty rooms available, and we can be close to each other that way."

Within the hour, the three of them were on their way, walking to the rooming house to retrieve Mardell's luggage, and then on to settle her at the Isle Hotel.

Finding this kind, friendly couple lifted her spirits. It was a blessing sent from God, to be sure. When Roger came in at nine o'clock that night, she was able to greet him with a smile.

One chilly day a short time later, Ken Kohler was walking to the hospital alone. He came upon a depressing scene. A streetperson, who had died that morning, was being loaded onto a stretcher. The body was dirty, unshaven, and the clothes were little more than rags.

A safety pin held a message, scrawled in crayon, to his jacket. Apparently written by the distraught "wino" as he realized he was near death, it read: "Use my body for any good cause."

His body was taken the one block to the Burn hospital. Later in the day, his skin was used on Ken's own son, Todd. Attached as a protective covering until they could use the child's own for grafting, it would remain on him for nearly a week. Then it would be "identified" by the child's system as foreign material and be sloughed off. By then the sheltered epidermas underneath would have had time to make itself ready for grafting.

No one ever found out just who the man was, or how long he had drifted on the fringes of society. They did know and would always remember, that he had bequeathed a vital part of himself for another suffering human being. His life had had value, after all.

And though he no doubt thought of himself as completely friendless in his final hours, there were many prayers that went up, prayers of those who could not have known his name. Prayers that petitioned, "Lord, have mercy on this poor man's soul!"

Each night before sleep, Mardell always included in her prayers: "Thy will be done. You gave us this child, so she is really yours. We want so much to keep her, but if you are going to take her, please do it soon, so she doesn't have to suffer any more. . . . ."

The first autograft surgery for Darla was scheduled for December 17. Because it was uncertain if she would survive surgery, Roger and the other children wanted to be with her the day prior. Ken, Judy and Roger took turns driving straight through from Iowa in 22 hours. They arrived in time for precious hours that might possibly be -- but they prayed would not be -- the last they would ever spend with her.

Darla's weight had dropped to a mere 17 pounds from her normal weight. Some days when her urine output was measured as only a few CC's, there was fear that she was slipping into renal failure.

During the wait for surgery to be over, the family paced the halls, round and round. The water fountain. . . .the elevator. . . .the restrooms. . . .the public phone booth. . . .the chairs and magazine racks. . . .and now to start again at the water fountain. When they could not walk any more, they sat and prayed silently.

In the operating room, the doctors were removing undamaged skin from her head and legs and applying them to her back. A machine called a dermatone was used to remove this first layer of skin. Because human hair roots are in the third layer, there was no danger of hair starting to grow in unwanted places on her body.

Before surgery her hair had been cut off and her head shaved. She would look like a little waif from a concentration camp for many weeks.

The nurses tried to prepare the family for her appearance when she would be wheeled back into the room. But it was shock nonetheless.

Her frail little body was lying stomach down with the new grafts on her back. The donor sites on her head were bloody, with layers of gauze to soak up and help dry the oozing blood.

A heat lamp was brought in to help the areas form crusts. In approximately two weeks, should she survive, the areas could be soaked off and then the site would be ready to be used once again.

Meanwhile the grafts which had been just laid on, had to be "rolled". A nurse with a sterile cotton tip swab would roll from the center to the edge to force out fluid that tended to build up from underneath. If not done, the new graft would not make good contact with the flesh and fail to grow together. It was uncomfortable for the patient, but not actually painful.

The day after Christmas was hard for everyone. Judy had to fly back to Iowa for school, her husband Jerry left to return to San Angelo, Texas, where he was now stationed with the Air force. And Darla was due for more surgery on the 28th.

This time it was to have steel pins placed in her heels for traction. The burns on her knees and groin area were pulling her legs up, a phenomenon known as contracture. Another submitting to total anesthetic. How many times could that little frame endure it?

Pat and Larry Dillonschneider, the parents of six-year old Matt, were from Kansas City. They became good friends with the Hansens, partly because they were staying in the same hotel. Like Roger, Larry had to go back home periodically.

Over the Christmas vacation, both families moved out to the the Sandpiper Motel on the beach, to take advantage of a place, where the children could swim and play. It was a relaxing and good therapy time for everyone.

A few days after Christmas, the temperatures plunged and there was a cold rain, bordering on sleet, which covered most of the state. After an exhausting day of visiting with Darla and activities with the other children, the Hansens went to bed early, and were sleeping soundly.

Just after 2 a.m., a fearful pounding on their door startled them to wakefulness. Roger staggered out of bed, knowing it must be bad news. He threw open the door to find Larry and Pat.

They brushed by him, into the room. "One of the doctors was just here," Larry said. "Matt died an hour ago."

As the Hansen children slept on, the four adults sat together at the wobbly motel table, drinking coffee and crying together. It had been so unexpected. It seemed as though the losses, the sorrows would never end.

It had been nearly dawn before they left the Hansen's room. Sleep was impossible now for Roger and Mardell. Together they watched the new day come.

Why had these other families lost their little ones and Darla still struggled on? Would they get a knock on their door some midnight, and be told that she was gone, too?

The following morning, the grieving parents and their remaining children, left with the body of their child, to return to Kansas City.

On New Year's Day Roger and the four children had to return to Iowa.

Mardell thought: I can't let them go back! I can't be here alone with Darla.

And more than once Roger asked himself: How can I go back and leave them here alone? But he knew that he could not put the whole burden of caring for the four children at home on Grandma Hoegh. He was torn two ways.

We'll take it one week at a time, they decided. God has given us the stamina so far, and if we trust Him, He'll continue to provide. On January third, Darla was turned on her back, after being on her stomach for 14 days. Her head was now out of shape due to neck contractions from having laid on the same side of her face the entire time. Again a shocking sight to see what appeared to be "half a head". This also precipitated an infection in the cartilage of her left ear.

It was determined that she needed a blood transfusion, and the only place available was into a vein in her already traumatized head.

Yet another surgery followed. Every scrap of unburned skin, except that which was on her head and still healing, was now grafted onto her stomach and left arm. A contracture in her left elbow was also released.

When she was brought back into the room, a pin had been set through her left wrist for traction to hold the grafted arm in the air. Her legs were also in traction, and it appeared as though the child was literally suspended in air from these three points.

After she was settled for the night, Mardell called Roger. This became Mardell's "lifeline". They shared their fears, their plans, and news from hospital and home. Tentative plans were for Roger to fly down whenever the home and farm situation allowed and a flight could be booked.

Mardell would tell Darla the plans, though she could never say the exact time he would come.

Yet on three separate occasions, Darla announced to her mother, "Here comes Daddy!"

Mardell would try to sooth her and assure her that, yes, he was coming soon, but was not here yet. Within half an hour each time, Roger would appear outside the room, smiling in at them from the window, before donning his special gown. It was as though Darla could feel her father's love was coming closer and closer.

One winter day as Roger stood staring out the window, he recognized a familiar pair as they made their way toward the entrance of the hospital. Leo Mardesens of Exira, Iowa were visiting a daughter and son-in-law in Pasadena, Texas, and had taken time to stop and see them.

It was so good to see someone from home! Harry and Lena Jensen of near Kimballton, also visiting relatives, stopped by. Later both couples were to tell them that though they were cheerful while visiting with Mardell and Roger, on the way to their cars, they broke down and cried.

Calvin and Phyllis Hoegh visited later. These three breaks in the depressing routine were a source of so much good will and sympathy, the Hansens were both bouyed and renewed, if only for a time. Also the cards and letters from home folks were so appreciated.

CHAPTER 5
DAY BY DAY

Roger continually pondered over what he could do to make life more bearable for Mardell, alone so much of the time, either at the hospital or motel.

"Let's go out for awhile tomorrow evening," he suggested during one visit. "I want to get you a TV so you can watch that in the evenings and try to get your mind off of things."

"I'd so much rather have a portable sewing machine," she answered. "That way I could get started on some spring clothes for the kids." She also thought of making something really special for the day that Darla would go home.

They ambled about a Sears showroom and picked out one that Mardell was to use for many years and still uses. It indeed provided a creative outlet for her and helped to shorten the long lonely winter evenings.

When he was back home in Iowa, Roger tried his best to keep things running normally for the rest of the family.

One Sunday sitting in church with the four children, he took a quick look in his billfold just as the organist started playing the offertory. The only bill there was a twenty. He wanted to give to the Lord what was His due. Yet at the end of the next week, there would be another plane fare to Texas. No other bills available, he slipped the twenty into the envelope.

The following Sunday, he was worshipping with Mardell in a Galveston church. Many of the members knew of the Hansen's situation, and there were many expressions of concern, as well as prayers. After services, as they walked out into the cool Texas air, an elderly gentleman patted Roger on the arm, gave Mardell an understanding smile and said, "It must cost a terrific amount for you to keep flying back and forth. . ." Roger thought he could feel something being put into his coat pocket.

As they walked down the street to find a cafe, Roger pulled out a twenty dollar bill. "Look, Mardell, I gave it to the Lord last week, and this week He gave it back!"

After a time, Darla was moved into a four bed ward. Each day's survival was a minor miracle.

The other three youngsters were also critically burned. A two-year old Spanish-American girl, a six year old Caucasian boy and a seven year old black girl were her room mates.

The schedule was such that from one to three in the afternoon was an enforced nap time for the children. The parents then usually went together for something to eat across the street from the hospital. In later years, they would be able to eat at the hospital. Now it was good to be forced to walk out the door into the fresh air.

In those two hours each mid-day, the parents became close friends, sharing each other's sorrow and worry. No two roommates were from the same state, but there developed a kinship that only comes with a shared heartache.

Twice weekly there were meetings for the parents. Either a doctor, physical therapist, social worker or psychiatrist led the discussion. It was informal, with plenty of chances for questions to be answered and anxieties to be put to rest. Sometimes a slide presentation would be given, showing in detail the reconstructive surgery.

One morning Mardell asked Dr. Larson (no relation to the hometown doctor) "How much reconstruction are we planning on for Darla as the months go by?"

The doctor put his hand on her shoulder, "Mrs. Hansen," he told her, "we aren't even thinking about that at this point. We are still just trying to keep your little girl alive."

It was a real blow for Mardell. She had felt after the first week in Texas that things had taken a definite turn and that there was no question that Darla would go home with them one day -- even though it might be months in the future!

Each day Darla would be wheeled to the whirlpool for debridement. All of the children, including Darla, hated this part of the treatment, because it was painful. Darla would sob silently as she spent her time in the water. But as the therapist helped her out, she would always murmur "Thank you."

As her burned areas became granulated, ready for skin grafts, homo-grafts -- skin taken from a human body other than one's own -- were applied. These homo-grafts were available from persons who had died at John Sealy Hospital and who had been compassionate enough to will their bodies to medical science.

The first and second degree burns on her hands and legs from her knees down, and her buttocks were healing now. There had luckily been no burns above her chin line, with the exception of one ear. Her thin little face was unscarred and her blond hair had been untouched. Third degree burns covered the rest of her body, the 85% which would need a slow and painful process of grafting.

By now several of the children who had been in the hospital before Darla came had reached a point in recovery so that they could be released. Others came to take their places, with new horror stories of the accidents.

As January crept slowly by, Darla was allowed to change positions one hour out of six. She was also started in the Hubbard tank for physical therapy. The next step was to put her on a tilt table. Very gradually, a few degrees at a time, she was introduced to the eventual upright position. So slow was the process that it took a total of four weeks. Following this, came the cautious trial of putting weight on her feet and legs.

On the 23rd Dr. Duane Larson brought the wonderful news that he at last had no doubt that Darla would survive. That date would be engraved on their hearts forever, as was the date of the accident.

Now came more surgery, this time to place autografts from Darla's head and the inside of her legs to repair her right arm and left knee cap. As January wound down, and on into February, there was one round of surgeries after the other, with Roger flying back and forth, trying his best to fulfill his dual roles.

On February 21, Darla was moved to a Stryker bed, which allowed her more freedom.

Later that week, the youngest child in the ward, the little two year old, died.

Roger had been in the hallway, just about to come into the ward, when Mrs. G., the mother, came out, staggering with grief. He saw at once what had happened.

Although they did not understand a word of each other's language, Roger instinctively began to comfort her. He put an arm around her and walked with her to the waiting room, where they sat, strangers sharing grief.

The next day, all of the parents who could leave, went to the Spanish service conducted at a Galveston funeral parlor. Then the little body was sent home, unaccompanied by the mother. The poor woman could not leave the Burn Center, for she had an older daughter who was also a patient there, having been burned badly at the same accident.

The two little girls, the younger riding piggyback on the older, had been playing in the yard, and as they happily jogged near a bonfire, an empty aerosol can exploded, spewing fire over both children.

Two weeks later the older girl died also, and the mother then returned home with the second body.

Mardell embraced Mrs. G. for the last time, offering words of comfort in English, which she just could not hold back, even though she knew the other woman could not understand her.

One word is the same in both languages, however. Mardell held her friend at arm's length and looked into the dark eyes so glazed with sorrow.

"Jesus," she said to her, and Mrs. G. nodded, even though the tears poured down her cheeks. "Jesus," she answered, forming her hands in an attitude of prayer.

This was their farewell. Mardell watched her walk, slowly, heavily, alone, down the hall to the elevator.

Each evening, before they left, Mardell would pray the Lord's Prayer as her last sharing of the day with Darla. "We have to leave, now, but Jesus is with you and will take care of you through the night."

One night, Darla replied, "But he can't get me a drink of pop if I get thirsty!" It was one of the few times they could actually smile, as they left her room.

"She has to be getting better, if she's making wisecracks!" Roger said. It made them both light-hearted.

Mardell had lived all her life in Iowa. A full-blooded Dane, living in Little Denmark, U.S.A., she had no idea what discrimination meant that year of 1967. She was soon to find out.

As Darla made progress, Mardell felt a need to get back to more regular Sunday worship. She told her new friend, Mrs. J., the black mother, "I won't see you until around noon tomorrow. I'm going to church."

Mrs. J. was also a Christian. "I wish we could go together," she said, wistfully.

"Come on, then," answered Mardell. "If we go together maybe we can figure out how to get there and back without getting lost!"

"Oh, I can't go to a white church, unless you find out first if it's OK."

This was culture shock for Mardell. In Iowa, blacks and other minorities were regular visitors in the churches, usually coming as part of a youth group or college choir, such as from Dana College, Waldorf College, or Augustana College.

"We'll get this straightened out!" Mardell assured her.

But it was not to be. Mardell thought by explaining that this woman was her friend, that they were going through a traumatic experience together, that they both needed Christian fellowship. . .

She could hardly believe that the pastor replied "I'm so sorry. . . .If it were up to me, it would be perfectly O.K. But you see some people in the congregation would not appreciate it. Not all of them, you understand. But some. "It just can't be done. . . ." He smiled apologetically at her.

"This is unreal!" she retorted. "I thought we were all Christians! Is this America?" In her emotional state, the tears, ever close, now glistened in her eyes. She turned from the pastor, feeling the stares of several of those nearby following her as she stepped outside.

Since the accident, neither of her parents had been allowed to hold or carry Darla, cuddle her, or have any sort of physical interaction. This was a frustrating part of the recovery. Any parent uses the blessing of touch to comfort and show love to a child. But because of the ever-present danger of infection to the burns, this was forbidden.

Her roommate now was a black child, Donna, just Darla's age. She was a wistful child, lonely much of the time, because her mother could not stay with her constantly, as could Mardell. Only her left arm had been injured, and since there were no other burns, she was free to walk about the room during her hospitalization.

One Saturday afternoon, while Roger was sitting by his daughter's bed reading, little Donna, shoving the book aside, crawled up on his lap to listen as well.

Roger put an arm around her to include her, giving her a smile and said, "I'm glad you're here."

Donna looked first at the book, then up at Roger. Back to look at the pictures, then admiringly up at this male parent figure. How nice, she probably thought, to have someone in my life like this!

As Roger paused for a drink of water, Donna piped up, "Will you be my daddy, too?"

Caught off guard, Roger glanced at his own child and then into the dark little face, looking up at him with so much longing.

"Well, it's this way, Donna," he answered, "besides Darla here, I already have five other children, and I guess that's about all the children I can take care of."

With a sigh of disappointment, she leaned back on his arm, to ponder over his reply. After that, Roger always tried to show extra attention to Donna.

Another day, and another story being read, and again, the question: "Won't you be my daddy, too?"

Before Roger could think up a better answer, or even repeat what he'd said the first time, Darla replied, "He already has enough kids of his own!"

When Darla was admitted to the Burn Center she was the first patient from Iowa. At that time the majority of the children were from the South. Space heaters used for homes were the cause of many deaths and dozens of accidents during the winter months. The girls would back up to the source of heat in an effort to get warm and their gowns would catch fire.

Had Darla been wearing pajamas rather than a gown she would have had even more extensive burns than she did have, for her legs would have had the material surrounding them, and the flames would have found their way as surely as dynamite follows the string attached to the detonator. Now government regulations insist on flame retardant materials. Darla's picture was used in pamphlets that were circulated throughout the U.S.A. to promote these materials.

Boys usually received their burns in different circumstances, such as throwing gas on a bonfire, putting gas in hot lawnmowers, spilling of hot grease in kitchen accidents, and vaporizers which tipped over, causing steam burns.

In one tragic case, a father tried to start a car by putting gas in the carburetor; a backfire ignited the gas, in reflex action he threw the can, and unknown to him, it hit the little son standing nearby. One incident, only hinted at, but confirmed later, involved a child who was purposely ignited by a mother, as punishment.

By the last day of February, a new plateau had been reached. For the first time, Darla actually walked -- in the Hubbard tank, the "walking tank" which helps the recovering patient relearn the skill by providing the buoyancy which only water can give.

LOOK magazine asked for permission to take pictures of Darla for a story. The Hansens hesitated, for they did not want to exploit their child. But if her story could give encouragement to those other children and their parents, it might be the right thing to do. The <u>Los Angeles Times</u> also took pictures and interviewed Mardell.

On the second of March, a stronger Darla because of the work in the tank, began walking on the floor in parallel bars at physical therapy. Mardell was surprised one afternoon when Darla came back into the room pushed in a wheelchair. Until then she had been transported on a guerney. Smiling at her mother from the wheelchair, she seemed less of a "patient."

More surgery was postponed, however, after Roger flew down, because a fever developed and a rash, the latter due to a reaction to medication. A compensation was that she now was able to roll herself front to back and vice versa, with no help.

When the surgery was at last completed, Dr. Larson came in on the third day and clapped his hands together to signal a forthcoming announcement.

"Now hear this!" he proclaimed. "Plan on taking this little 'fighter' home at the end of the month!"

Tears of joy and laughter this time. It <u>was</u> going to have a happy ending, after all. Mardell's heart was lighter than it had been for months. She and Roger watched Darla ride a tricycle determinedly in a wobbly circle about the therapy room.

At last -- they had left the valley.

41

CHAPTER 6
PREJUDICE

A dying person in need of a heart or kidney transplant cares little who the donor is. It little matters if he was young or old, Catholic, evangelical, charismatic, or of whatever ethnic group.

Most burn patients, while awaiting the time that they could receive their own autografts, gladly accept homografts from whatever is available.

But not all. The children of course are too young to have learned prejudice. Some of their parents or guardians do have decided antipathy towards accepting anything other than from white donors.

One of the little girls was wheeled back from surgery sporting several black homografts. Her aunt-guardian was aghast.

"What have you done to her?" she demanded. "Take that black skin off of her this minute!" She was almost out of control.

The nurse hurried out of the room to find the doctor. Luckily he was at the nurses' center, getting ready to follow up on his little patient.

He explained as quietly as he could, "Mrs. A.," he began, "this was all that was available. You should consider your niece lucky that we could find this. She badly needs this -- and now. Without them, it will be even more of a problem to keep her body fluids from escaping."

"Well, I simply won't have it!"

"What do you suggest? That we wheel this dangerously ill child back in there, remove them, expose her to infection..."

"My skin! Take my skin!" she screamed. "But get that -- that <u>stuff</u> off of her -- or I'm removing her from this hospital!"

The doctor looked at her for a long moment, weighing the child's dangerous condition against the very strong desire to tell this unreasonable women what he thought of her.

"All right," he said. "It's forcing her to undergo another anesthetic. It's your choice!"

And so the aunt's donor skin was removed. But afterwards she became very ill, and had to remain in her own room, not visiting the child for several days.

In the aunt's custody, with no father or mother to sit by her bedside, the little girl grieved for her aunt, not understanding why she had been left alone, why yet another adult had failed her. Rapidly, her condition declined. She seemed to have given up. Within the week, she died.

The other families were deeply saddened and greatly angry by the needless loss. They felt it had been an unnecessary sacrifice to the aunt's biased ideas. The child had been the innocent victim.

Darla was covered with black skin at one time and that probably helped save her life. Pig skin was also used on patients.

CHAPTER 7
ANOTHER LOSS

As Mardell sat reading to Darla one day, a nurse came into the room and asked her to step into the hall. The nurse's pretty face showed that she was the bearer of bad news.

"Carmelita just expired," she told her. "The mother really needs someone. I know you two can't understand each other, but maybe you can help her."

Mardell hurried down the corridor. She had heard yesterday that the child was failing fast. There was no chance of recovery, and very heavy medication was necessary in order to numb the excruciating pain.

Mrs. L. stood outside her daughter's room, sobbing out her grief. They walked into the room, Mardell's arm supporting the other woman. The bed where her little one had laid for so long, in such agony, she now lay upon in peace. All of the life supports had been whisked out of view.

They stood by the bed, for a last look before the funeral director would wheel her away.

"Mi nina," Mrs. L. moaned, "Mi nina es muerte!"

Mardell laid a hand upon her shoulder, as the mother looked up at her. There was gratitude that this other mother had left her own child's bedside to come to her.

Despite the fact that Mrs. L. could not understand Mardell's English, Mardell spoke to her slowly, comfortingly, speaking of a God who loves us, who sent his Son, Jesus, who has a place for us in Heaven.

And she could tell from the response, her nodding, her growing calmness, that this suffering mother understood the message, if not the language in which it was spoken. Mrs. L. touched the cross she always wore about her neck, and managed a weak smile.

"Jesus," she repeated, and folded her work-worn hands in an attitude of prayer.

They said their farewells. Sisters in Christ, bound together in a faith that was shared, even though it could not be articulated.

CHAPTER 8
KAPTAIN KWIK

There was a bonding among the parents. Spending time together daily, several times a day, facing the same uncertainty regarding their child's life or death, the continual witnessing of the children's agony, wove these people together in a way that no other friendship could ever duplicate.

Backgrounds were dissimilar. Rural and urban, poor and middle-class, one parent and two parent, Christian and non-believer -- all thrown together because of one common experience - a child's burns.

When visiting hours were over at eight P.M., a group which varied in size, would walk together to the Kaptain Kwik sandwich shop, close to the hospital. If some of the fathers were there, there might be as many as a dozen. Sometimes one couple or another elected to just skip supper and go back to their rooms to munch apples and write letters home.

Each one tried to keep up the spirits of the others. They tried to find bits of humor to lighten the gloom. Pet names were chosen for some of the hospital staff, which provided a few needed laughs.

Other patrons of the shop would have no idea that the members of the jolly group were all parents of children who were so critically ill at the Burn Center. They appeared to be just a group of friends having a bite to eat before going to a movie.

The meal and conversation provided a badly needed outlet after a day of intense worry.

CHAPTER 9
GOODBYE, TEXAS

As they readied themselves to leave the hospital, emotions became mixed, swiftly changing, and bittersweet. There was happiness because of going home, at last. But there was also a reluctance to be saying goodbye to the new friends, the caring nurses and doctors and therapists.

Some of the patients and their parents would never be seen again. Before the Hansens returned for a scheduled check-up in August, several of the children would be dismissed and their paths would never cross again.

Before leaving, Darla was fitted with a blonde wig. The stiff lining irritated her healing scars and she made one of her few complaints. "It hurts me and tickles me at the same time!" She would pull it off every chance she got.

Later at home at a church service, she tolerated it until the pastor started reading the announcements -- then off it came. She was, at four and a half years, more interested in being comfortable than appearing stylish.

A special spoon was sent along for use at home. It had an extra long handle to accommodate getting the food to her mouth when her underarm contractions made it difficult.

Purple was Darla's favorite color at the time, and the coat and bonnet Mardell made were that color, a pretty compliment to the pink Easter dress. At a therapist's suggestion, a pattern was chosen that could be altered with snaps all the way up the middle of the back, necessary since Darla was not yet able to raise her arms.

While still in the process of preparing for the move, 1000 miles north in Iowa, there was vicarious rejoicing for Darla and her family. The <u>Des Moines Register</u> reported her return in three different editions of the paper. Pictures of Darla, smiling in her new spring outfit accompanies the feature.

Donald Kaul's column, usually sardonic or witty, was uncharacteristically tender in its tribute to the courage of the entire family.

And in "Over the Coffee," Gordon Gammack, who was to later write a book on his coverage of three wars and his interviews with service men and women so gallantly serving our nation, this day devoted his space to a tiny little Iowan who did not realize how close she had come to death, or how many Iowans had been remembering her in prayer.

Suitcases were packed and the new sewing machine in its case. Good-bye now to Lzetta Halingstad, the Norwegian mother from Montana. Her little son, Lars, had received serious burns on the top of his head as hot grease from the stove spilled on him as he sat in his stroller.

Lzetta's husband, Harold, had spent much time in the hospital and the two families had become very close. This friendship was to flourish over the years, and visits to each other's homes have been enjoyed.

Gene Griffith, another good friend, came to the motel early to help Mardell with the luggage.

Darla was excited and happy, decked out in her new finery. Her thin little legs were wrapped in elastic bandages and her feet thrust into slippers. Gene accompanied them to the airport, and his strong young arms carried Darla onto the plane.

Gene was the evening receptionist at the Burn Center, whose daylight hours were spent as a medical student at the University of Texas. He had a genuine love for people and tried in every way to provide support for the patients and their parents.

His tie with the Hansens was to continue through the years and he was to visit them several times. They, in turn, paid him a return call in 1984 at Troy, Montana, where he now practices medicine.

As they left Texas that Good Friday, nearly $30,000 had been spent on Darla's care. Not a significant sum by today's inflationary standards, but in that day a monstrous amount. Friends -- and strangers -- had contributed a total of $1,700 for travel expenses for the parents.

Darla sat, wide-eyed and quiet as the jet's engines whined and the travel attendants made their pre-flight checks up and down the aisle.

A stewardess stopped to speak to her. "Well, young lady, are you going on a trip, or are you going back home?"

Very seriously, Darla looked up at her. "I'm going home," she answered. "I've been gone too long!"

A light and gentle rain was falling on the parched Iowa earth as the plane banked to approach the Des Moines Municipal Airport. The Midwest's drought was growing more serious by the day. The Des Moines fire department had answered an unprecedented 138 fire alarms on Friday and in Council Bluffs there had been a total of 24.

Now the break in the dry spell seemed a further omen of a change of luck, not only for Darla, but for the whole state.

Waiting for them at the gate were Roger and the five brothers and sisters and Judy's husband, Jerry. But not only they! Several Shrine representatives were on hand, and the Shrine clowns were there to liven things up, presenting Darla with a huge stuffed Easter bunny.

Other passengers arriving in Des Moines, and those on hand to meet them, delayed their own departures to watch the joyous scene. Many a stranger brushed away tears, perhaps thinking of a small child in their own life.

Flash bulbs went off continually, as state and local papers recorded the event for the next day's editions.

On the way home, Darla, Connie, Lori and Jeff sang "Here Comes Peter Cottontail!" even harmonizing as they loved to do. Waiting for them in the yard was Grandmother Hoegh, laughing and crying and urging them all to "Come in! Come in!" A good hot supper waited them. "All the things that Darla likes."

But once the prayers of thanksgiving were over, at least one chair was empty throughout the meal. Each of them had to take turns answering the phone, which seemed to ring constantly with good wishes and "Welcome back!"

After 135 days in the Shriner's Hospital in faraway Texas, they were finally home.

CHAPTER 10
HOME AGAIN

On Easter Sunday a family dinner was planned at Grandmother Hoegh's. She had been away from her own kitchen so much since early November that she was anxious for a chance to get back and prepare a huge holiday meal for her children and grandchildren.

Izy Hoegh, Emery's wife, felt it might be necessary to prepare her own Carol, then five, before the family gathering. She was afraid that Carol might blurt out something about Darla's scars that would hurt her feelings.

She sat down with her, before leaving for the dinner, trying to explain how Darla would look different, but would be the same old Darla, who was not only cousin, but fast friend since they were babies.

Returning home that evening, Carol leaned over from the back seat of the car. "Mama, I thought you said Darla would have rough skin. Her skin wasn't rough."

Izy felt a tightening in her throat. She pressed her lips together, and watched the countryside go by, outside the car window.

"Oh, if we could all look at each other with the eyes of a child" she thought. "If we could just see the real person as they do. . . ."

In the meantime, Lori, being next to the youngest, was feeling an understandable resentment of all the attention coming to Darla. It seemed that it was always "Darla this..." and "Darla that..."

She wanted to shout "I'm here too!" At seven years old, she couldn't reason that she was no less loved than she had ever been.

On Easter Monday, Lori was pulling Darla in a little wagon. "Stand up, Darla," she coaxed. "It'll be more fun if you're standing up!"

Innocently, Darla brought herself to a standing position. Lori took off at a trot, Darla fell out of the wagon as planned, and the result was an injured arm, cracked in two places. She wore a sling for two weeks, when X-rays showed that it was healed.

Connie, too, had been feeling the stress which the whole family was under. In January, when semester grades were given, she had received an "F" in junior high typing, because she couldn't finish her assignments in class.

There was no typewriter at home. Others in the class were able to stay after school to work on assignments. But because her parents were in Texas, Connie had to ride the bus right after school. If they had been home, they would have told Connie to stay, do her work, and then wait to be picked up at Grandmother Hoegh's house, right across the street from the school.

But Grandma was at the Hansen farm, babysitting. And all because of Darla. The family was revolving around Darla and her needs.

Connie hated the "F". No one in the family had ever gotten one before. She had stared out of the bus window as she rode home on the day report cards were handed out.

"It's not my fault!" she thought.

CHAPTER 11
ADJUSTMENTS

Darla was still far from being well. Her home care took up a great deal of time. Each day began with Mardell supervising Darla as she sat in the tub for thirty minutes. Then, as they became ready Mardell removed the scabs.

With the natural inclination of a child her age, Darla yearned to be active. But most activity required a great deal of effort for her. As she struggled to get into the high chair, it would have been easier to just lift her in. Instead, she would hear, "That's the way, Darla. Yes, put your left foot further over towards the leg of the chair. Good girl!"

Judy, with her nurse's perspective warned against doing too much for her, so that she would become self-centered and spoiled.

"She's going to have enough to battle, with her scars," Judy warned. "If she turns into a spoiled brat, people will have one more reason to turn away from her."

Often she would totter and fall while walking across the room, awkward with her legs wrapped, and the constant "pull" of the healing wounds. But if she lost her balance and fell, she soon knew that she was to crawl to the nearest footstool or chair or table and pull herself upright.

It was so hard to ignore her and continue to fold towels, stir cake dough, do homework, or figure out a new ration for the cattle. Sometimes whoever was closest to her in the room would have to turn their eyes away, steeling themselves not to rush to her, knowing it was for her good.

"She's going to have to do a lot of this on her own," the doctor had said. "And you are going to have to let her." And with each incident, she did grow stronger and more adept at handling herself.

At the living room doorway, a long narrow paper was taped, showing how far Darla could reach. As she attained one goal, the marks were inched ever higher.

Included in her home therapy routine, was a simple exercise to train her right thumb from its stubborn tendency to contract back toward the wrist. Several times a day she would be reminded to tuck her thumb into her palm and hold it there.

It became so much a part of the daily pattern that she soon did it without being told, and over twenty years later, she still finds herself doing her "thumb tuck."

What a blessed relief it was for Mardell to be back in her own home again. Here were husband, Lori, Connie, Jeff and Ken -- and Judy only an hour away. This was her nest. No more wanting an item of clothing, a sewing notion, a favorite book, only to know that it was at home in Iowa and not in the gloomy hotel room.

Here was her own bed, stove, phone. And within reach, the extended family, neighbors and friends. As she moved about the kitchen the first full day at home, running her hand appreciatively over the counters and seeing the familiar housekeeping items again, she breathed a prayer of thanks.

Her mother had left everything so spotless. And there were baked goods in the freezer which she had prepared, and some that had been brought in by friends and neighbors.

But, conversely, it was an emotional shock to reorient herself after the long winter of stress. For five months, all of her waking hours had been spent at Darla's bedside, as comforter.

Now she was to be the primary care-giver, with no backup of the skilled nurses and doctors and therapists. She felt terrified at the responsibility. And she felt guilty at feeling this way, and trying to hide it compounded the anxiety.

In addition to her nursing duties, she now had the household tasks, which she had been away from so long.

Each time that Roger rose from the table to attend to his farm duties, she felt a flush of abandonment. "How long do you have to be outside?" she would ask.

"Do you have to go to town this morning? Couldn't it wait until the kids are home from school?"

I'm not a nurse, she thought. _What if I'm upstairs and Darla needs me? What if. . . ._

One afternoon while Darla was napping, she sat at the kitchen table. "Lord," she prayed, "you were with me all those months at the hospital. I could feel the support that could only have come from You. Help me now that we're home and I feel so burdened."

She sat quietly for a time, meditating. Her strength had not come from the doctors and nurses! They were the ones who said now was the time to go home. Other people needed their time and attention now. And, thanks be to God, Darla had reached the point where she no longer needed to be in the hospital.

There seemed to be a lightening of her load. She would be given help each day, for each new challenge. As she got up, to resume her household duties, things seemed to have been resolved.

The family eased into a routine which involved Lori and Connie taking turns being with Darla in the period between school and supper. Cooking and baking duties were made lighter by the casseroles, pies, cookies and whole meals which came in from kind and generous women in the community.

Once in a while, Mardell stole half an hour for herself, to tramp about the farm, breathing deeply of the good Iowa fresh air, the scent of the grasses and clover growing. She watched the cows with their new calves, peacefully grazing, the sheep on a neighbor's hill, so far away they looked like patches of clouds that had drifted down from the sky.

Thoughts cleared and tension drained from her body at such times.

As she walked about, in her old comfortable chore boots, her stride took on a rhythm that seemed to accompany a prayer she had said hundreds of times since the accident: "Thank you for bringing us <u>this</u> far, Lord . . .Thank you for bringing us <u>this</u> far!"

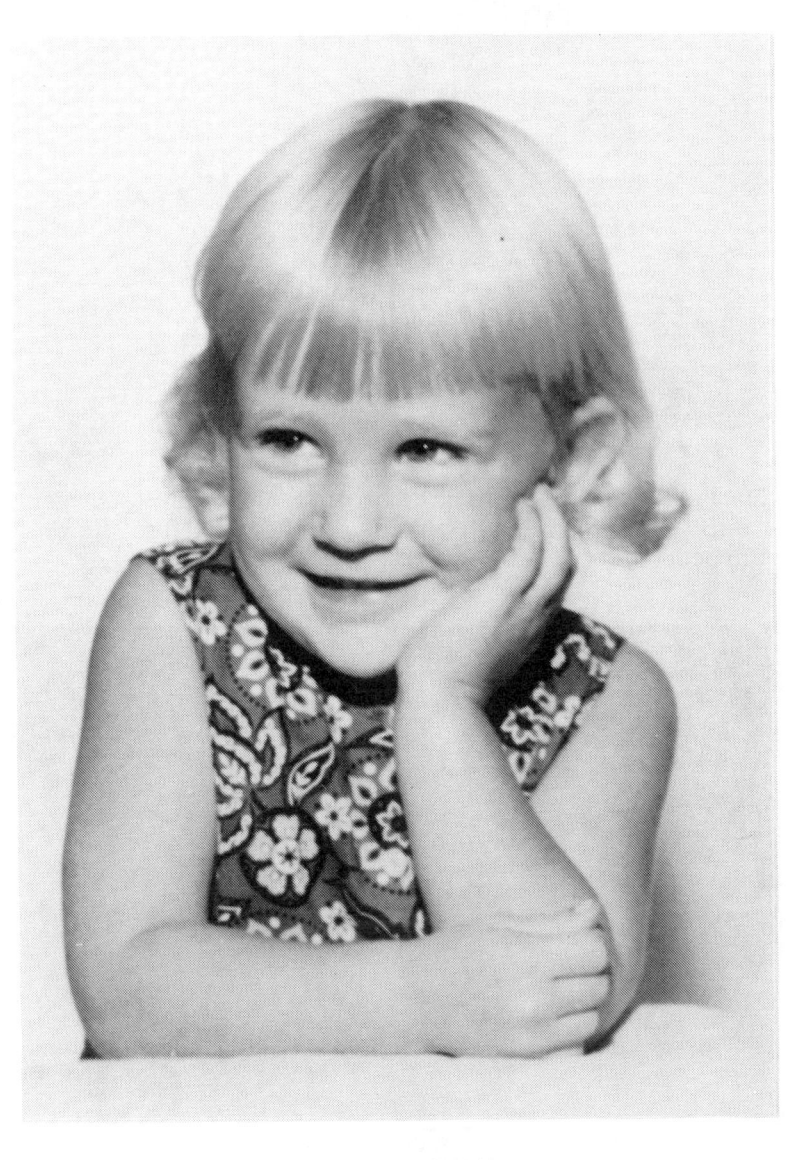

Darla age 3 1/2.
This was taken the summer before the accident.

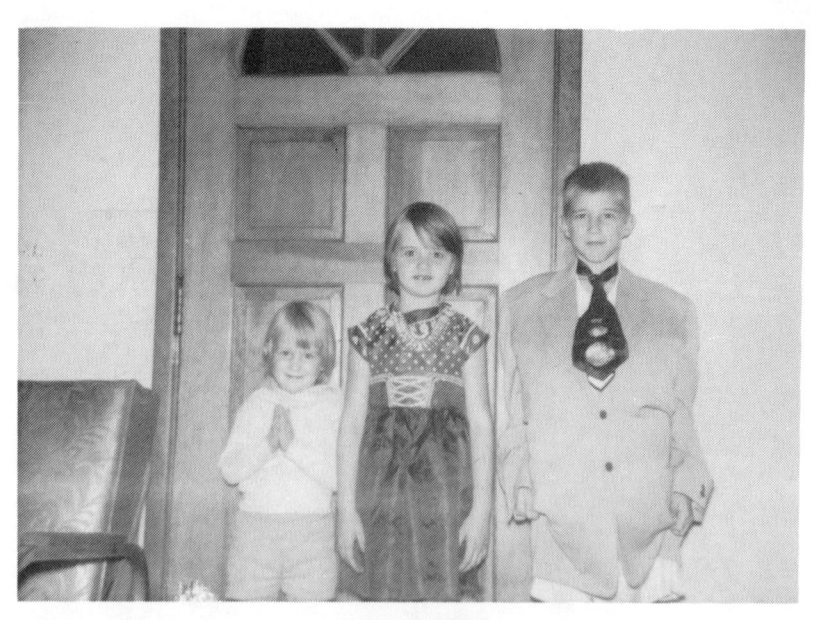

Darla with sister, Lori and brother, Jeff, on Halloween 1966. This was her 4th birthday just days before she was burned.

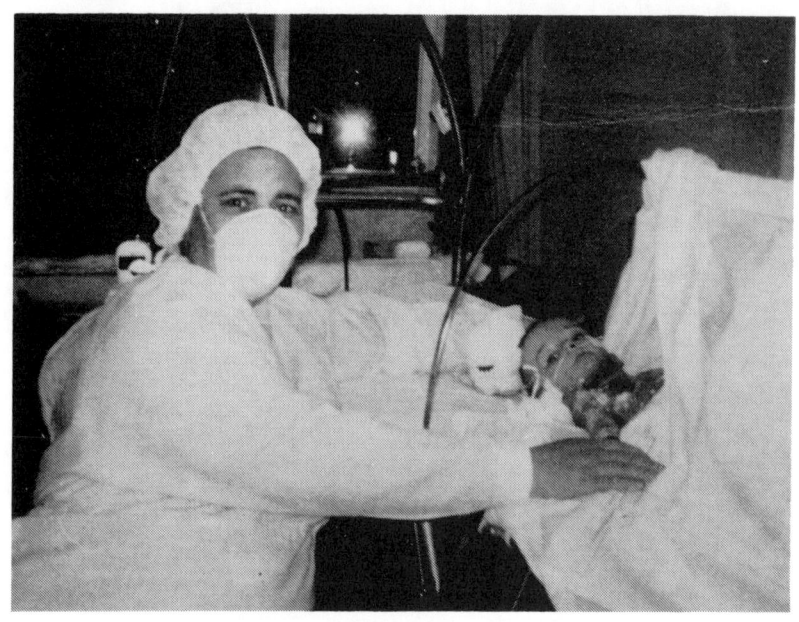

Darla with her mother. Darla has a feeding tube in place to assure she was getting proper nourishment.

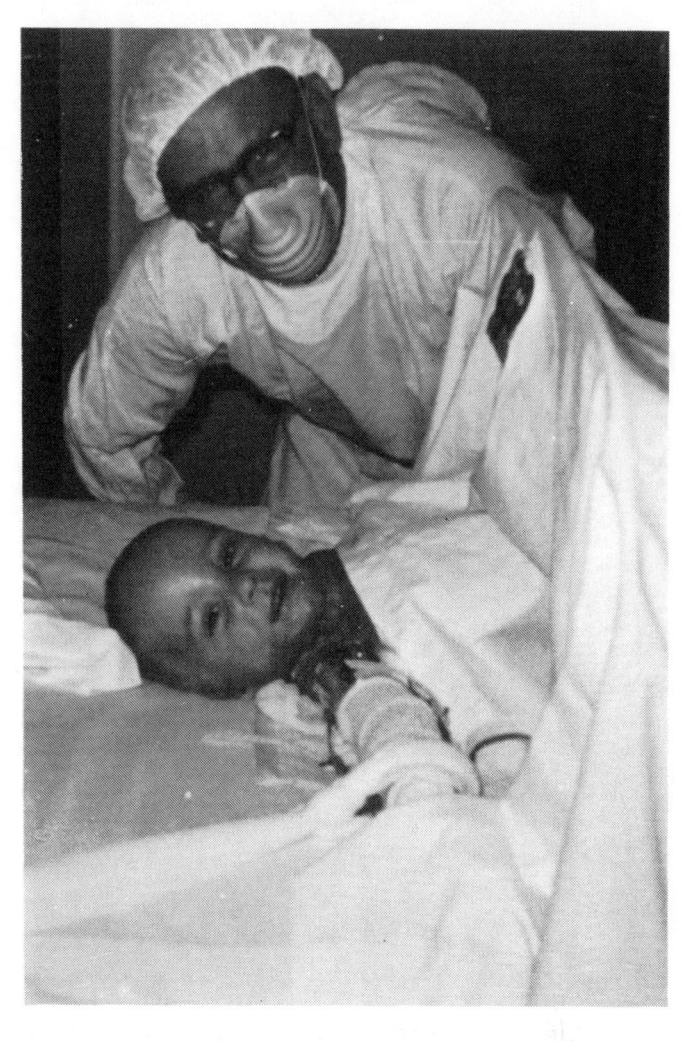

Darla with her father. Visitors were required to wear gowns, masks, hats and shoe coverings to avoid possible contamination. Items brought in to Darla had to be sterilized in an autoclave.

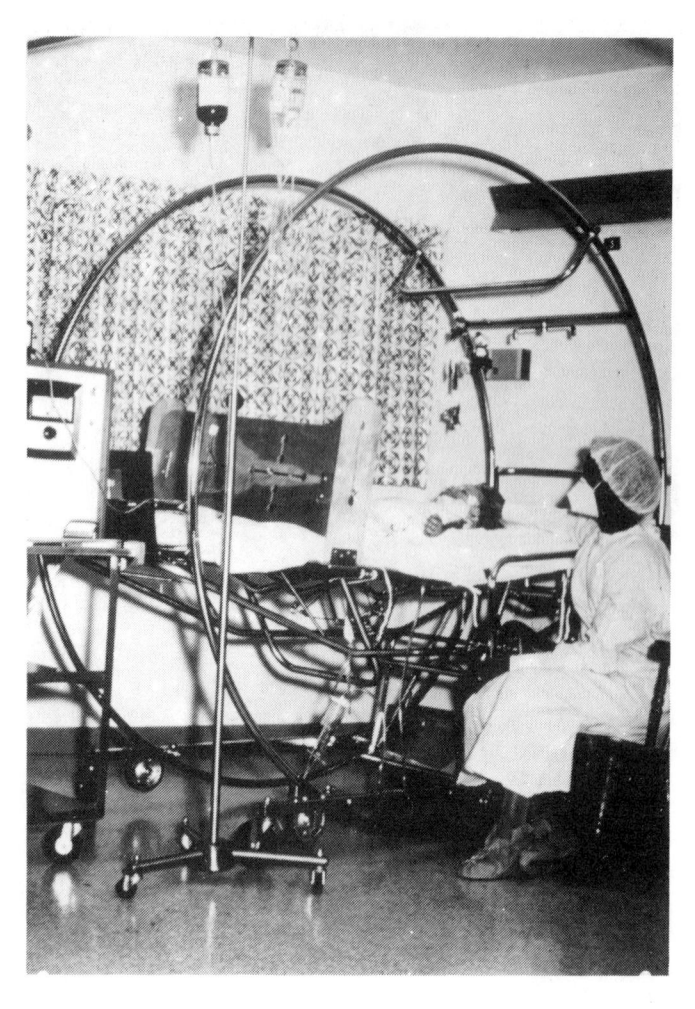

Darla in a circular electric bed hooked up to monitoring equipment that records temperature. As temperature changes a thermal blanket is warmed or cooled.

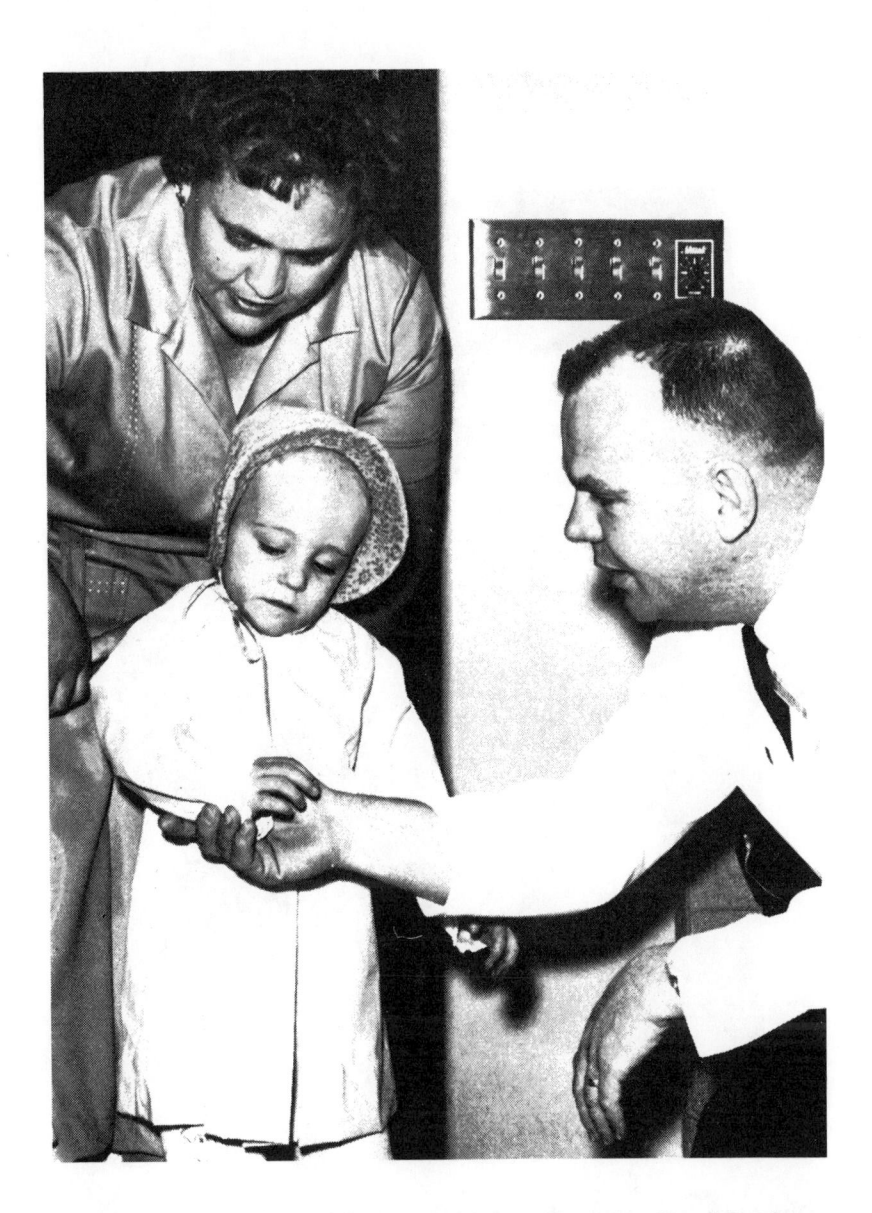

Darla, her mother and Dr. Duane Larson on Good Friday the day of Darla's dismissal from the hospital. It was appropriate that this was the 1 year anniversary of the first admissions to the Shrinier's Galveston Unit. Darla was the largest burn that had been salvaged to date.

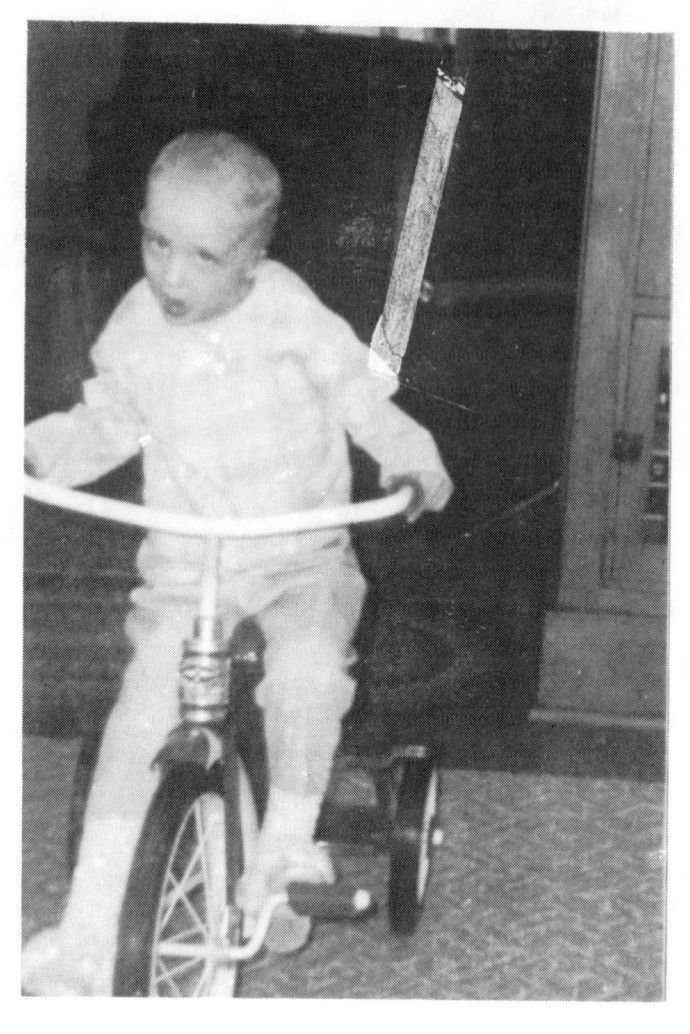

Darla on her new tricycle within 1 month after returning home from Texas.

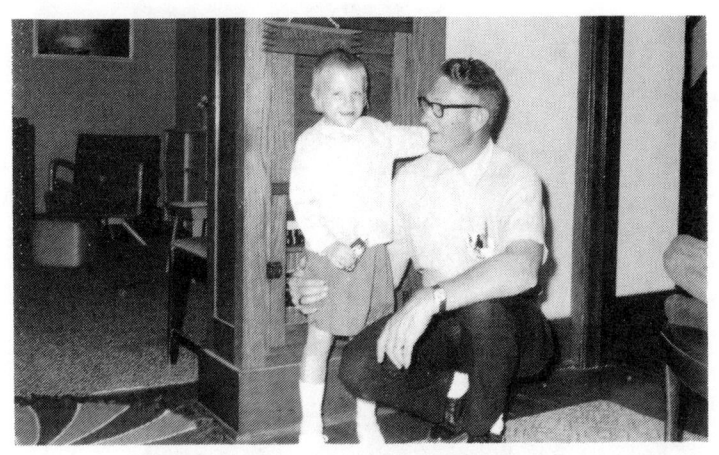

Darla with Shrine Dad, Howard Juel, of Kimballton. This was 1 year after critical burns.

Flammable Sleepwear

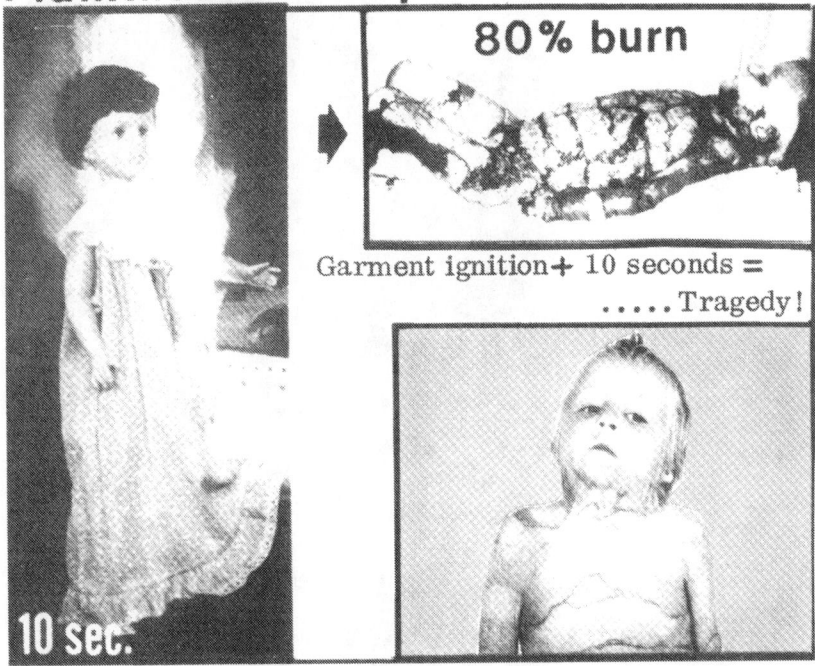

80% burn

Garment ignition + 10 seconds = ... Tragedy!

10 sec.

This was a pamphlet the Shriners circulated throughout North America to promote a bill to be passed requiring flame retardant sleepwear. The 80% burn photos shown are of Darla.

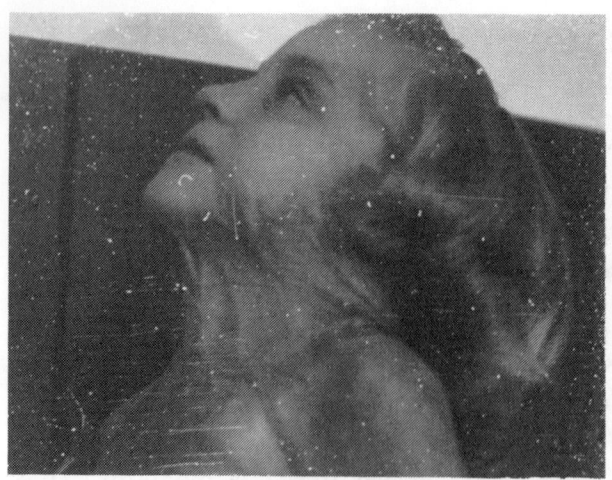

Darla at age 7. Some reconstructive surgery had already been done on her neck, but more was needed.

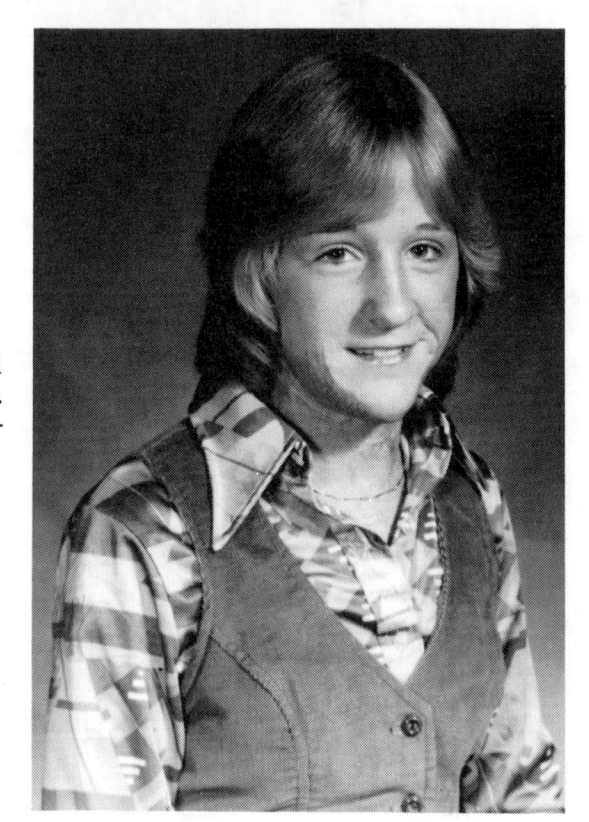

Darla's school picture from Jr. High School - age 14.

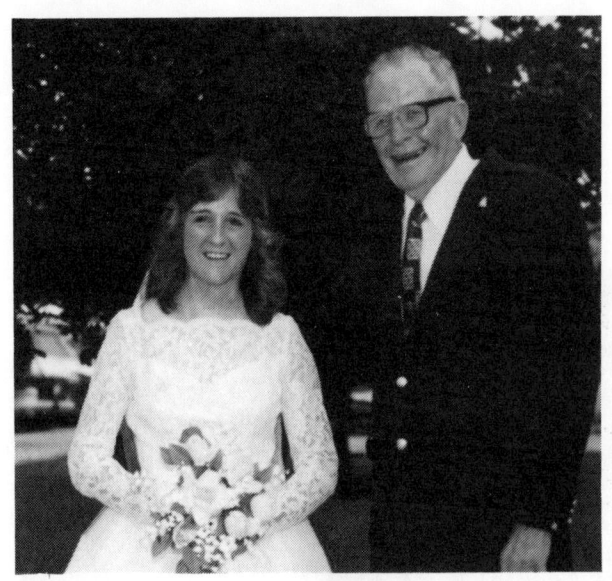

Darla with Ted Cutler on her wedding day August 8th, 1981. Ted was Shrine Potentate the year Darla was burned and became a lifelong friend.

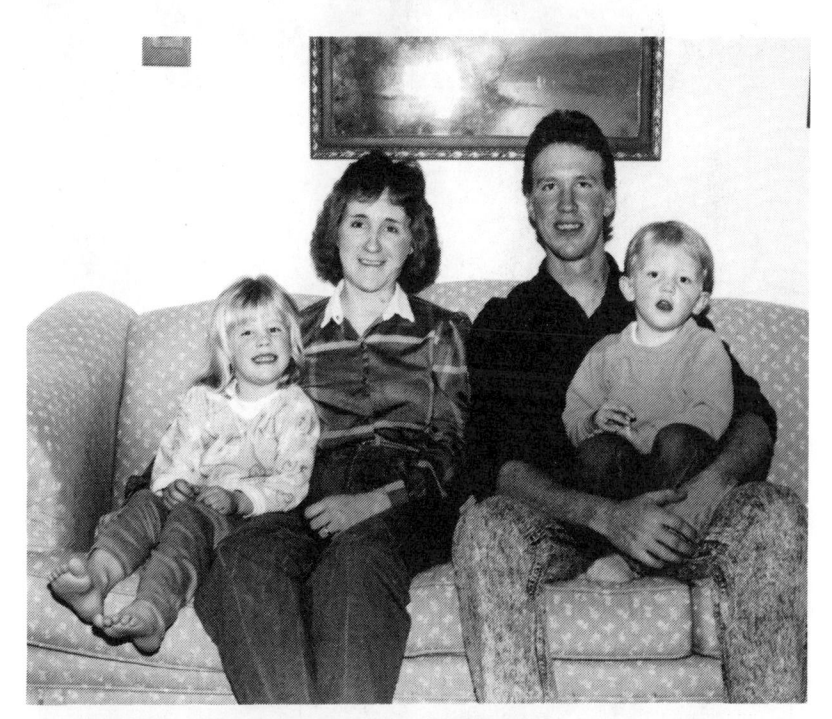

Darla with her family in 1990. Daughter, Monica age 4, husband, Derek, and son, Jordan age 3.

Family picture 1989:
front row - Judy, Lori & Connie;
middle row - Mardell & Darla;
back row - Ken, Roger & Jeff

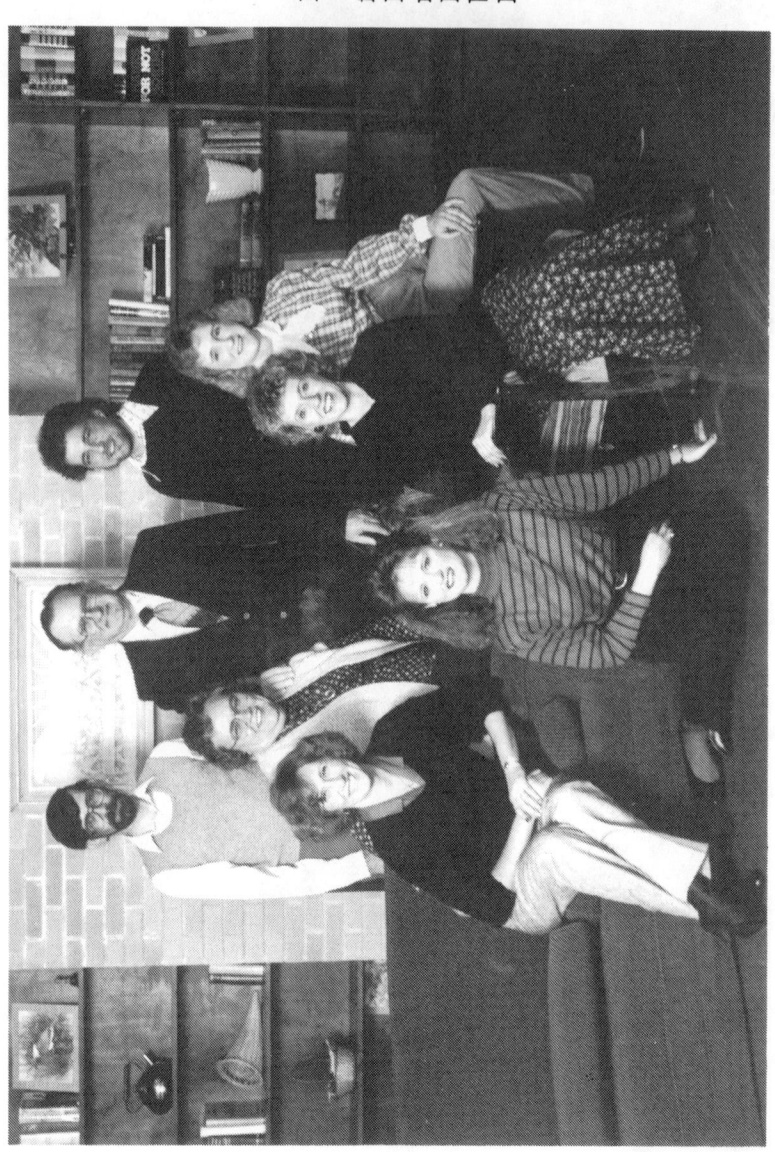

To Darla

A sweet little girl only four years old
Got badly burned one day
But she coped with her scars and went on to help
Other people to go on their way
So, lets give a clap to our therapist now
And wish for her only the best
She gets tired, I know, but goes diligently on
In spite of needing a rest.
       Mable Mutum, 1990
       Resident, Salem
         Lutheran Home

Here we are in Galveston
Darla, Rog' and me
We're many, many miles from home
Yet your faces we can see.

We always will remember
How kind you've been to us
Although you may not know it,
It's meant so much to us.

The Shriners are so gracious
To care for Darla here
Facilities are tremendous
They have all kinds of gear.

Oh yes, there are some nurses here
To mention one, there's John
When it's time to give the medicine
Oh! Oh! That John is gone!

Of course there's Womack and Mrs. Clark
They come from Texas City
Clark is tall and sweet and kind
Womack's right-down pretty.

I have a friend named Francis
She comes from Biloxi
Although she is a colored girl
It makes no diff to me.

You see she's been here long as I
Her girl, Debbie is six
She's in the bed right next to Dar'
Now see --- "All races mix".

I also have another friend
And her first name is Pat
She lost her boy last Saturday
That Darling, little Matt.

She went back to Kansas City
With a heavy, heavy heart
It's just so hard to understand
Why loved ones have to part.

Now Darla is some better
The doctors all are glad
We thank the Good Lord Daily
For the Part that He has had.

That Mrs. Latham, she's a doll
Real peppy, no not dull
If there's nothing really important to do
She'll just "Shoot the bull".

Then there's Miss Willson, me oh my
How I wish she liked me
I know when one o'clock comes round,
But, <u>she</u> reminds me daily.

We have a woman doctor here
Abston is her name
This lady is remarkable
<u>Prediction: "Hall of Fame"</u>.

Down in the lobby, behind the desk
"This happens to be on first floor"
There sits a chap, his name is Gene
He'll say Hi! as you come in the door.

From the pan-handle of Texas, Gene says he comes
And he's proud of his town you can bet
A nicer Texan you'll never find
At least, I <u>ain't</u> found one yet.

Darla's been so very brave
She doesn't hardly cry
You say, "We'll get her well again?"
Lord knows, "We're going to try!!"

              Written by Mardell Hansen
                    January, 1967

CHAPTER 12
MOVING ON

So many gestures of goodwill revealed the caring nature of the large community. From the Atlantic Rainbow Girls came a new tricycle. The group had asked the Hansens for a suggestion for a gift, and the three-wheeler would not only be a source for fun, but good therapy, too.

Darla loved to be outside, after so long a time of constantly forced to be inside. But outdoor play had to be monitored in the warm months, as sunburn would have been disastrous for her. Her arms were to be covered at all times, to prevent even a superficial burn.

Her parents took a more relaxed attitude than the doctors, and at the first return trip to the hospital in August, Darla was sporting a healthy suntan, with no obvious adverse effects.

That first year, and for many years thereafter, the Hansens were given a generous amount of Shrine Circus tickets, which they shared with friends. Howard Juel, Johnnie Westphalen and Johnnie Jensen were instrumental for arranging this.

The Iowa Shriners also had a midsummer party at Camp Sunnyside near Des Moines for all children from the state who had received treatment at the Burn Center. At Christmas time a special luncheon was held with gifts, entertainment, Santa Claus and food.

which provided yet another time for fellowship and fun for those having a common experience.

A once-in-a-lifetime thrill was experienced at the Shriners Night at the Shrine Auditorium in Des Moines. The famous Wayne King orchestra was presenting a concert. At intermission, Darla was introduced to the packed house as having just returned home from a lengthy hospital stay. Howard Juel, Darla's Shrine Dad, walked out onto the stage, holding Darla's wee hand. The moist-eyed crowd exploded into applause.

"Do you have a favorite song, Darla?" the famous band leader asked.

"Winchester Cathedral", she answered, without any prompting. The audience chuckled at her rather sophisticated choice, and the orchestra obliged. To cap the evening, Mr. King gave her an autographed picture, which she carried home to add to her growing mound of treasures.

Each time Darla was taken someplace again for the first time since coming home, it was more traumatic for others than for her.

Her first visit to the local bank with Mardell was a pleasant one for her. One of the tellers chatted with her and gave her the customary balloon.

As they finished their business and started out, Jim Jacobsen entered. An elderly retired farmer, Jim knew the Hansens well, for the older children had been accompanied on the piano by his wife, Mayme, for instrumental solos in inter-school contests. Darla had often tagged along when they practiced. Jim remembered her from before the accident as active, normal, happy and pretty.

Now, her still-healing appearance struck him like a blow. He wheeled about, fighting tears, and stood on the sidewalk outside.

The friend, Gene Griffith, medical student and receptionist from Galveston and a friend, Jane, stopped one day at the Hansen farm. As Darla ran toward him, as any normal child would at seeing a well-liked visitor, he remembered how he had thought after the accident that it really would be best if Darla died! Now it seemed so unfair for him to have even thought such a thing.

At her tender age, Darla of course had no conception at the enormity of what had happened to her, or of how it would forever affect her life.

One day, playing with cousin Carol Hoegh and sister Lori, Lori asked, "Darla, would you rather be burned and have all these toys--or not be burned and not have the toys?"

Coolly, Darla looked about the room which did indeed have a great many toys, games, stuffed animals and other gifts that had been sent or brought by well-wishers.

"I'd rather be burned and have the toys," she decided. And seriously continued her task of the moment--giving her new stuffed Teddy Bear his candy mint "medicine."

In late April the local school held its annual fund raiser Fun Night. Sponsored by the P.T.A., it involved a cake walk, food booths, and a variety of entertainment. When the Hansens arrived, with Darla in tow, it was one of the first outings they had had, apart from church and family gatherings, since coming home.

Most of their acquaintances greeted them warmly. Some made it a point to speak to Darla, some seemed ill at ease and avoided looking at her.

One thoughtless person asked rudely, "Why did you bring her?" *Her*, not Darla, as if she could not hear. Roger was so shocked he could not reply.

Holding her hand, he turned away into the crowd, hoping to find something to divert Darla's attention. Why had they brought her? They had brought her because she had wanted to come along and because they were proud of their youngest, just as they were of their other five children. They had not guessed they would be ridiculed for having her at a public gathering.

CHAPTER 13
PHASE TWO

In August the return trips to the Burn Center began. They could not know at the time that they would be continued for over thirteen years, until Darla was seventeen.

Judy was on summer leave from training and she and Ken were left at home to do the farm chores and keep house. Mardell and Roger started out with the other four children.

On the way, they stopped at Neosho, Missouri, to spend the night with the Brasiolas, whose son Rocky had been a fellow patient of Darla's.

Another stop-over was always at Mardell's brother, Dale and his wife, Jean, in Ft. Worth, Texas. Darla remembers one such stop we rode the shortest subway at the Leonard Bros. Department Store and Dale and Jean bought her a cowboy hat. Uncle Dale thought she should have a traditional Texas hat.

Once at the hospital, the first order of business was to shave Darla's head once again, as her hair was sprouting up willy-nilly between the scabs.

Then: six more surgeries. Skin was removed from her right leg and grafted onto her neck so that she could once again have a defined chin line. Also repaired were her left arm, left thumb, groin and heels.

Placed on a double mattress, her head was then positioned to hang over the edge of the top mattress in order to stretch out the neck and allow for healing without wrinkles.

This resulted in a continual headache for several days. Her spirits remained good, however. She would reply with cheery remarks, when asked how things were going, despite eight days of not being able to move her head or neck.

When she was finally able to walk, the doctors fitted her with a neck brace to hold it rigid. This she would have to wear for six months, the latter half of the time only at night.

This time the family had pulled a house trailer behind their car and parked near the beach so that the other children could enjoy the beach during the long hours one or both parents would be at the hospital.

Shortly after they arrived in Texas, Dean Petersen, a twelve-year-old neighbor boy was admitted. He had been initially treated in Omaha for burns suffered in a tractor accident. His mother, Ardis, stayed with the Hansens the first night of her arrival.

The two families lived only a few miles apart. It was a cruel coincidence that both young families should be devastated by burn accidents.

Dean was treated in the first wing, which is reserved for "fresh" (new) burn victims. Darla had stayed there the previous winter. Now she was in the second wing, where "old" burns were reconstructed, old scars reduced, and increased mobility achieved, through surgery and additional instruction in therapy.

The family started back home on the 25th, despite the fact that Darla had developed a kidney infection. A prescription was sent along and within a few days, the problem was cleared.

But in September, she succumbed to a bout of pneumonia. A hospital stay in Harlan was necessary. Once home, all was quiet for two short weeks, at which time, Darla fell while playing and ripped out a graft under her left arm.

"What next!" Mardell wondered on the hurried trip to Dr. G.E. Larson.

As he stitched the graft in place, he admonished his small patient, "Take it easy for a while, Darla, please!"

But she did not follow his advice. While lining up "goodies" for one of her innumerable tea parties, Darla decided to have a pre-party snack and nibbled down 25 baby aspirins. Back to Harlan to have her stomach pumped!

At the end of February, 1968, another trip to the Burn Center was scheduled. Darla was now past five years old, and weighed a very slight 45 pounds.

As a reaction to the pain she had endured, she had so ground her baby teeth together, that they had been virtually worn away. She had no permanent teeth. Dentist Paul Emmert James, a cousin of Mardelle's, of

Audubon, Iowa made her some false teeth to fill in the gaps. Her medical records note that she had scoliosis of the spine, with a tendency to the right. This later corrected itself.

On this trip surgery was done to release old scars and to make a new graft on her right arm.

CHAPTER 14
SCHOOL YEARS

In rural communities where children see each other not just in class, but at church, 4-H meetings and at neighborhood gatherings, they become so used to one another, that one accepts the others without thought of anything deviating from the norm.

Darla recalls very few times when she received thoughtless or cruel taunts about her scars. Once, though, in fourth grade, a couple of her classmates came up to her at recess and teased her about her looks. The remarks continued the next day, as the boys could see they were getting to her. It cut like a knife to Darla. She had known them all of her school years. Why were they starting this?

The elementary counselor, Carl Cochran, handled it wisely and told her that those particular people were just showing how immature they were. He suggested she make a retort about their haircuts--nothing mean--but enough to make them stop and think that everyone perhaps has something about them that doesn't look so great to others. The next time one boy tried to send a wounding remark her way, Darla replied as suggested. End of the teasing!

Just before a surgery in July of 1977, one of the social workers came in and brought a cassette tape which was intended to relax her and put her in the right frame of mind for the ordeal.

The following morning, Darla thought she would give it a try. A female voice on the tape began in a soothing tone, talking about ocean breezes and sitting by the ocean on a lovely summer day.

To Darla, groggy from the pre-surgery hypo, the drone of the voice combined with the narcotic to made her nauseated and she rang for the nurse to stop the tape. She drifted off quietly, then, ready for yet another operation.

After so many, many times being wheeled into the cold, green operating room, Darla began to have a real aversion to it and even had bad dreams concerning that room.

As Darla matured, she came to appreciate her parents more and more. She realized that her accident had been a turning point in family life--that financially it had added a great burden, that the trips back to the Burn Center had been the focal points of family plans for many years.

Yet never had she heard, or even sensed, anything negative from either of her parents. She felt nothing but love and support from both of them. Having parents like she'd been blessed with was a gift from God. The older she became, the more she realized how lucky she was.

One of the memories she carries is that of Mardell struggling to turn her heavy hospital bed so that Darla, still groggy from the anesthetic, could see the television which a roommate was watching. "The

Brady Bunch", one of her favorites, was flickering across the screen.

"That day is so vivid in my mind," she recalls. "Mom moving that heavy bed, trying to avoid all the attachments, doing anything and everything to make me happy. My eyes were blurry from still being sleeping and the ointment they put in your eyes in surgery to keep them from drying. I lay there, batting my eyes, trying to be awake, trying to watch the program, but after about five minutes I fell off to sleep. Mom would never complain, though. Day after day she did so much for me. . . "

CHAPTER 15
THE SOUND OF MUSIC

Music was interwoven into the fabric of Hansen family life.

Judy has said, "If Dad wasn't listening to the markets or weather on the radio, he had Big Band music on his stereo. I thought then that was what every household was like, but I know now it was just us, and it was great to be exposed to so much good music."

Mardell adds, "Roger and I still play organ and drums together and Roger still has music playing a big percent of our day, and even in our bedroom at night."

She had been blessed with the gift of playing the accordion and organ by ear. This ability and the enjoyment she and Roger shared, instilled a love of music in all six of their children.

Judy played clarinet and saxophone, Jeff the trumpet and French horn, Ken sax and guitar, Lori, the flute. Roger had a set of drums that he taught himself to play. By the time Darla was in fifth grade, she chose the saxophone.

During the time Jerry was courting Judy, he was impressed by the way the family enjoyed making music together. At Christmas, more time was spent in singing and playing religious carols and secular holiday music than on gifts.

Music played an increasingly important part of Darla's life.

In third grade, the elementary vocal music teacher recognized the quality of her voice and picked Darla to sing "O Holy Night" in the Christmas program.

The children's choir at the church was another chance for Darla to sing. Twice the group performed on <u>Miss Jean's Story Time</u>, a Christian T.V. Sunday morning program, on KMTV in Omaha.

Her friend, Janell Sorensen (Hansen) and Darla both played the saxophone and the girls vied with each other for first chair in the band. Darla then switched to the tenor sax and the problem was solved, giving the band more depth as well.

When they were still in eighth grade, both girls were honored by being asked to play with the high school jazz band.

CHAPTER 16
LESSONS

At age 10, when Darla was in the fourth grade, it was time for reconstructive surgery on her left ear. By this age a child's ears have reached the size they will be as an adult, and there was no reason to delay longer.

Before checking in at the hospital, it was necessary to go to an optometrist and get a non-prescription pair of glasses. Using the earpiece as a guide, the ear was reformed. On the earpiece was a hard cast shaped like an orange slice. This kept the "new" ear from growing flat against her head.

Typically, Darla found this an occasion for humor. "See my new specs?" she would ask. "I had to get them for my ear."

"Say--what?"

"Repeat that, please!"

"Come on, Darla! Glasses for your ear!"

The surgery included placing a synthetic hard center in the upper part of the ear. When she "pings" it with her finger, it makes a musical noise. She enjoys showing this to new acquaintances as a part of explaining her accident.

The optometrist who fitted the glasses and made sure she really did not need a prescription pair, did not charge for them. A Shriner himself, Dr. R.L. Smith of Atlantic, Iowa, was happy to be a part of the recovery team.

On one return trip to Texas, Darla and the other youngsters were taken to the hospital playroom to meet someone "special." The kids were anticipating someone to entertain them or to talk to them about their own experience.

But the young lady who met them was special in a way that made their own problems seem minor. For she was, in addition to being an unusually short person, one who had been born without arms, only flipper-like appendages joined to her shoulders. Yet she had her own apartment and was employed.

She demonstrated how she could type and comb her hair using her feet. Some of the youngsters reacted with remarks such as "Oh, it's gross!" or "I can't stand to look!" or "Why did they make us come in and look at <u>that</u>?"

But Darla was impressed. Her conclusion was that probably each human being must have a handicap of one sort or the other. Some are of course more visible than others.

Two years later, another trip to Texas, this time only as an outpatient. Wonderful not to have to stay!

She could always see the humor in her situation. Sometimes after returning to Iowa, she would have to have stitches removed. Brother-in-law Jerry would do the honors, and she would then tell people she was being treated by a Veterinarian!

Contact was maintained with several of the friends Darla had made at the hospital. There were the three Brenda's--from Mississippi, Louisiana, and Texas, and Lars from Montana. As they grew older, the Louisiana Brenda, Steve, and Darla would try to plan to be back in the hospital at the same time. They were now the oldest of the returnees, and liked to think they were "in charge."

Much of the time was spent visiting and playing with the younger children.

One year, after surgery, Darla contracted staph infection from one of the little ones and was immediately put in isolation. With no visitors allowed, it was a depressing time for her at first. But soon Brenda caught it also and was moved in.

One of the young nurses, knowing the girls needed a lift to their spirits, helped Brenda and Darla sneak down to the employee cafeteria and get each of them a candy bar. The entire furtive adventure took less than five minutes. But it provided some much needed giggles and the feeling that they had some control over things.

Over the years, the letters from Brenda have dwindled and contact has been lost. Steve, who was originally from Georgia, is married and was at this writing in his residency at the University of Texas, as a surgeon. He had always vowed he was going to be an anesthesiologist at Shriner's Hospital.

Two others whom Darla enjoyed were Solidad, a girl from Panama, with whom she exchanged letters for a few years, and Tami, a Mormon girl from Utah.

Darla enjoyed sports in junior high, was a starting guard on the basketball team. The following spring, she placed well in high jumping during the track season. In eighth grade she won a coveted first place in high jump in the Western Iowa Conference. She also was a member of the relay team, running 220 yards or less. Her only restriction was the caution regarding overheating.

As a freshman, she went out for basketball, but did not make the varsity. Again going out for track, she pulled a leg muscle and had to quit.

A southpaw, Darla went out for softball and was a natural at first base. She earned a varsity suit and played in a few varsity games.

In July of 1977, the summer before she would enter high school, she was once again in Texas for surgery.

The second day after reconstruction, June, a favorite nurse, came in with a huge package. She kicked the door shut with one foot and grinned at her patient.

"What are they sending you? I'm surprised this thing got through the mail!"

"Open it, please," Darla whispered.

"Always prepared!" June answered and whisked out her nurse's scissors. The box was open in seconds.

A huge white polar bear, stuffed and beribboned, held a greeting card between its two paws. Coach Taylor and the entire softball team had signed their names and added encouraging messages. They knew how disappointed she was to have to miss practices and games in order to make her trek to the hospital.

"I'll put him over here," June said, plunking him down on the dresser. "And if you don't take your medicine he's going to report to me!"

Darla drifted off to sleep, smiling at June's remark, thinking how great it was to come from a small town where people cared, and kept caring, year after year.

The doctors reemphasized the precaution about no sunburns and no over-heating. Sunburning leads to peeling and that would precipitate more scar tissue. The absence of many of her sweat glands made it hard for her to perspire normally. Her head, buttocks and right leg are the only parts of her body which can get rid of waste in this manner.

But with care, she had handled it. She had even gone on an extended bike trip with her pal, Janell Sorensen. One day she did have to give in to warning signs and rode in the car for two hours.

Dave Taylor was the softball coach the first two years she played summer softball. The father of three, the youngest of whom was handicapped, Taylor was a sensitive and caring teacher and coach. When he announced that he and his family were moving on to a larger school, the whole team was "down".

They dreaded to think of just who would be hired to follow him. None of the local teachers had the time to assume this additional position. A man from out of the community was hired, and from the first day, it was obvious he considered himself a top sergeant in the U.S. Marines, rather than a coach of teenage girls who were playing ball for the fun of it.

One July afternoon, the team was practicing at five in the afternoon, to accommodate girls who had summer jobs. The temperature hovered at a deadly 95 F. Darla arrived at practice after working at the local grocery store.

After about 45 minutes of working out, she felt herself overheating. Her face turned a dangerous florid.

Jana Petersen, a friend and teammate suggested she sit down on the bench. Immediately the new coach stormed over to check. Darla started to explain.

"You see, I have to watch out. . ."

"Do you want to play ball this summer or not?"

"For medical reasons I have to. . ."

"Why you think you are somebody special I'll never know!" he hollered, not listening at all.

Jana came to her defense. "Darla doesn't think that, but when she was little she got burned and. . ."

"You keep out of this!" He turned a livid face to Jana and jabbed a finger in the air in her direction.

Neither of them could make him understand. He would not keep still and listen.

"You're soft! That's all that it comes down to! Soft! You kids get spoiled at home and then come out for ball and think everyone else is going to stand aside for you! You sit at home all day in air conditioning watching T.V. and then come out here and you can't take it, can you?"

He seemed to enjoy his own performance. He stomped back to the field. The girls exchanged looks and shook their heads at his unreasonableness. Darla had the urge to leave right then.

"I'm not going to give him the satisfaction of leaving now, though," she told Jana. She finished the day's practice, thankful for clouds that gathered which minimized the sun's impact.

After practice, she turned in her suit. It was a big disappointment. But she was now old enough to know she couldn't let her love for the game endanger her health and she knew he did not understand her situation. It was a sad day for her.

CHAPTER 17
MOVING--WITH RESERVATIONS

Elk Horn was home to Darla. She knew everyone and was known and accepted by everyone. She could go anywhere--church, school, activities, the park or swimming pool and not have to feel shy or do any explaining about her scars.

Then half way through her sophomore year everything turned upside down for her. Mardell and Roger sold their farm and bought a house, retiring to Atlantic.

She thought she just could not leave her friends, some of whom she had been with since the first day of school.

Judy and Jerry were now situated four miles south of town as Jerry had a vet practice in Elk Horn. There was some discussion of Darla living with them for the last years of school. But the out-of-district tuition would add up to thousands of dollars.

Sadly, she accepted the move. Here I am, she thought the first day going into the new high school. Here I am, big as life. Here's Darla, scars and all. What you see is what I am. And by the way, what have you got to show me?

Her friendship with a few Atlantic teenagers helped. And friend Jody had introduced her to the Salt Cellar, the Christian youth center in the downtown area. Now she would be able to use it more, and it would serve as a center for broadening her friendship base.

In the basement of an appliance store, the Salt Cellar is a nondenominational Christian Coffee House for young people. It affords a wonderful chance for the youth of the area to meet and fellowship with others who want to relax and have fun apart from the drinking and drug scene. Each Saturday night features a Christian musical group, speakers or movies.

The Now Disciples was a gospel singing group comprised of six high school students and a number of young adults. Darla loved to hear them and enjoyed the special witness in song. When an opening, due to a graduation came, Darla tried out for and won the spot.

This afforded her a chance to really gain self-assurance in front of an audience. Darla started giving her Christian testimony. Each time, she spoke of her accident and made it clear that God was the healer.

During the year the Now Disciples performed throughout the area in churches and in concert. Each summer they went on a tour for one or two weeks. The summer before Darla's senior year, they traveled to Estes Park, Colorado for the annual Christian Artist's Camp.

The group was thrilled to see and hear such great artists as Amy Grant, B.J. Thomas, Evie and others. And through the daily Bible study, they increased in knowledge of His Word.

She had hated the idea of moving. Yet one good thing seemed to unfold for her after another.

Around the first of February, a graduating senior quit her job at HIS Bible and Book Store on Chestnut Street, the main street of the business district. Darla applied to the owner, Fran Cornwell, and was accepted. Fran became a friend as well as her boss.

Each night after school she would work for an hour, until nine o'clock on Thursday nights and on Saturdays. It was a job, but it was also a joy. Most of the customers were Christians. And it provided a great opportunity to keep up on the latest Christian books and albums. Darla was to continue working there off and on until she finished her nurses training.

Within weeks of enrolling at the new school, Darla won a position in swing choir. But nothing ever seemed to be simple for her. It was as though this new cause for happiness and being accepted had to have its price.

Getting ready for the first concert, the members were building a human pyramid. Darla fell and sprained her left ankle. It was more painful than when her arm was broken as a child. Crutches were in order.

But she was used to pain after all the months at Galveston. This was minor. She toughed out the dance routines the night of the concert, putting on a smile for the audience and concentrating on them and the steps, rather than her own discomfort. She could handle a <u>sprain</u>!

After the fire, anything she would ever have to go through could be handled. She seemed to have gained a stoic acceptance of pain, a mature grasp of duty beyond her years. And she knew from whence came her strength and courage.

CHAPTER 18
DEREK

A year after moving, Darla had increased her circle of friends, through school, church and the Salt Cellar.

It was there she had met Joel Hansen, and when she was invited to his seventeenth birthday party at his home, she was to meet his younger brother, Derek, with whom she later fell in love.

Her previous dates had all been on a casual, friendship basis. With Derek, it was "special" from the start.

He was just a year ahead of her, and as a senior was thinking ahead to college. After the party, they greeted one another at school, but nothing more.

Then one September Sunday, Darla was part of a group singing at the Emmanuel Baptist Church, which Derek's family attended. Milling around after services with other young people, they found themselves on the fringe of a jovial, kidding group. It was almost as though they had both maneuvered to stand close to the other.

"What are you up to this afternoon?" She could hardly believe she'd blurted it out.

He grinned down at her "Washing my car." He had a '69 green Roadrunner, which Darla considered one of the neatest cars at school.

"Coincidence! That's what I've got to do. Come on over and we can do it together!" This was not really in her plans, but sounded like a good way to spend the afternoon with Derek.

"O.K.," he agreed. "I'll see you after we've had dinner."

Two weeks later they attended the Homecoming dance together. And from then on, there was no one else for either of them.

From the first, they had serious discussions about Darla's scars.

Repeatedly Derek told her, "If the scars bothered me, I wouldn't have started dating you in the first place!" And then he would kid her that of course they were destined to be married. She wouldn't even have to change her last name!

A sobering consideration was that of children. There was a real possibility that because of the scars across her midsection and abdomen, Darla might not be able to carry a child.

It was very possible that there was not enough elasticity to allow for the growing and stretching that accompanies pregnancy.

She could believe him that the scars were of no consequence. But not to have children of their own! And she so much wanted to be a mother some day. He assured her now that it would not matter. But what about later? Would adopted children make up to him for not being able to hold his own flesh and blood in his arms?

No one brought up the idea of not having children to Derek. But many times friends or relatives would ask him if it didn't bother him when strangers would stare at them in the city shopping malls.

He always snapped back, "She's a lot better person for going through what she's had to, than those rude people will ever be!" What other people thought was of no concern to him. It was their problem, not his.

Long before Derek's family met Darla's, his mother, Marilyn had prayed for Darla. Prayed that her life would be spared, and that she would suffer no permanent disabilities from the accident. Now, more than a decade later, it appeared that this little girl had grown up to be the girl her son Derek would marry.

Darla made her last trip to Galveston alone. The summer before her senior year, and now 17, she felt she could make this last journey with no parent along for support.

This time, minor surgery was done to release scar tissue on her left shoulder and left knee.

It was strange--almost sad!--to think that she would never be coming back here as a patient. This had in a real sense been her second home. Her care had been marvelous. Not only had the staff saved her life, but their extraordinary skills had rescued her from a life as a crippled and perhaps wheelchair-bound person.

Her life was full, happy, wonderful. And she was now old enough to realize these people were largely responsible for it being so.

"There is no way I can say 'thank you' enough," she told the staff. "You've done so much for me. . .so much. . ." There were hugs all around, moist eyes, and a reluctance to at last say farewell.

As she boarded the plane to return home, Darla had the thought that this was very much like a graduation. Almost 14 years of flights back and forth, of surgeries and therapies, and now it was over.

The plane rose into the Texas-blue sky. "Goodbye, Burn Center," she spoke softly as the city fast disappeared below her. "Goodbye, and thank you."

She relaxed against the seat. "And thank you, dear Lord, Maker, Redeemer, and Healer. . . ."

Derek was on hand to pick her up as the plane touched down in Omaha. He understood that she would be having mixed emotions about this last trip.

He entered into the post-operative care of her stitches, applying the hydrogen peroxide, and even removed her stitches on the appointed day.

CHAPTER 19
CHANGE OF PLANS

Following high school graduation, Derek began attending college at the University of Iowa.

Thanksgiving, with Derek on vacation from the university, meant a few precious days together. The night before the holiday, which they planned to spend split-time with both families, they talked constantly of how wonderful it would be when Darla graduated at mid-term, joined Derek in Iowa City, and began her own training. No more expensive long distance calls or too-short weekends with the 400 mile round trip drive.

The next day, after church, Derek drove out to see his maternal grandparents, Arnold and Erma Westphalen, at their farm home near Elk Horn. Plans were to have seen them that evening for a buffet supper at his parents. But Grandfather and Derek needed to talk about Derek's interest and desire to farm.

The elderly man and the young one walked now about the place up into the pasture where the stock cows still found plenty of late fall grazing.

By the time they returned to the house, Derek was ready to burst with excitement. His grandfather had offered him a chance to farm with him, starting the following spring. It had been what he had always dreamed of, despite being a town boy. It was literally a dream come true.

He finished out the semester, but as he was later to admit, spent most of his time at the library doing research on hogs and their various diseases!

Plans for college were also altered for Darla. With Derek gone from Iowa City, she had no interest in the program there. Instead she registered at Iowa Western Practical Nursing Program, working also as a nurse's aide to help with expenses.

CHAPTER 20
WEDDING BELLS

The dreams and plans meshed in the perfect day, with everyone Darla loved around her to share the happiness of the wedding day.

On August 8, 1981, not quite fifteen years after the accident, she walked down the center aisle of St. Paul's Lutheran Church on the arm of her proud father. Pastor Rothfusz of the church and Pastor Hoover from the Emmanual Baptist of Atlantic served as joint ministers.

To include everyone that deserved a special place in the wedding party, it turned out to be a moderately large affair, with four attendants for the bride and groom.

Jody Andersen (Stevenson), for whom Darla had been maid of honor the previous May; Jody, the neighbor girl who had so faithfully walked over to play and share tea parties and later teenage confidences, was matron of honor. Lori and Connie, Darla's sisters, were bridesmaids, as was another friend, Jan Wolfe. They all looked fresh and lovely in the wedding colors of peach and silver.

Derek's friend, Jeff Gipple, was his best man, with his two brothers, Tom and Joel and pal, Kelly Simonton as groomsmen.

Judy, Darla's oldest sister, and Derek's aunt, Karolyn Ortgies sat at the guest book table.

As they were planning the wedding, Darla asked if it was O.K. with Derek if she sang. "That is, if I don't get stage fright -- or start crying!"

Derek agreed that this would be more than appropriate.

And so brother Ken joined Darla in a duet just before the bridesmaids walked down the aisle. When the first chords of the Wedding March rang through the church, tears welled up in Darla's eyes. She looked up at Roger and bride and father looked deep into one another's eyes. He covered her trembling hand with his.

What a long fifteen years it had been! And now to have it end so happily. Someone gave Roger a gentle shove, and they started down the carpeted aisle.

As the wedding party stood before the altar, Deb Fields, vocal music teacher in Elk Horn, and active at the Salt Cellar sang "He has Chosen You for Me." Janell Sorensen, another school friend from since before kindergarten was organist. Kim Petersen, friend and also Derek's cousin, played "Trumpet Voluntary."

It was a real celebration of love and happiness. But there was a specialness not usually found at a marriage ceremony. For here, too, was a triumph of courage and stubbornness.

So easily could the bride have withdrawn herself from society. So easily could she have retreated into self-pity.

Later, Mr. Ted Cutler, a Shriner from Des Moines, who called himself Darla's adopted grandfather told them: "It was the most beautiful wedding I've ever been to--bar none! I've been at the Crystal Cathedral in California when Roger Williams, the great pianist, was married. Robert Schuller performed the ceremony. But this tops even that!"

Honored guests were Grandfather and Grandmother Wesphalen and Grandmother Hoegh and husband Hans. P. Hansen.

At the very end, a comic note was added, due to the pastor's microphone remaining on. After saying, "I now pronounce you man and wife," and smiling at the announcement, there was an awkward silence, for he had forgotten the words about kissing the bride.

For a few moments nothing happened and then Darla's voice: "We're supposed to kiss now!" It blared out over the whole church. As Derek bent down to oblige, both he and Darla were chuckling as were most of the people in church.

There was no immediate honeymoon. After the reception, the newlyweds drove slowly up to the little rented house near Rorbeck, for their first night as man and wife. The following evening, both families joined them in the fun of opening the gifts.

Several weeks later, between job demands and preparing for Darla's schooling, they squeezed in a two-day honeymoon in Des Moines, shopping and attending the famous Iowa State Fair.

CHAPTER 21
SETTLING IN

Nurse's training began in September. Gayleen Sornson, a close friend from Elk Horn was also enrolled in the Licensed Practical Nurse course.

The work and school days were long. Derek worked at a factory in Atlantic besides farming and started work there at seven in the morning. The young couple rose before daylight, the chores were done at the Westphalen farm, and the 12 miles to Atlantic were driven. Derek, getting off at three in the afternoon would then wait for Darla to finish her class and they would then drive again to do evening chores, eat, relax a bit, and fall into bed by nine o'clock.

One of the nurse instructors told Darla that if she felt uncomfortable wearing her hair up off her neck, she would not hold her to the regulation. Darla thanked her for her concern, but with a few rare exceptions decided to follow the rule.

She was chosen class president while in training. She helped field the complaints from other students, was among those planning the capping ceremony, and gave a short speech at graduation.

After graduation, Darla worked nights as charge nurse at the Salem Nursing Home in Elk Horn for a year and a half, followed by six months at the Anita Nursing Home. She appreciated the day shift, but returned to Elk Horn to start a rehabilitation therapy program for the patients. She had received training for this at Myrtue Memorial in Harlan, where she had been taken first following the accident.

This combination of being a nurse and therapy assistant fulfilled a desire to help others as she had been helped.

And now her thoughts turned again to the possibility of motherhood.

A local doctor recommended that she visit a prominent plastic surgeon in Omaha. It proved to be a discouraging afternoon. He maintained that the only way she could carry a baby to full term was to have reconstructive surgery to release a couple of binding scars on her abdomen. He was insistent that she should schedule for the following week.

Darla felt pushed and uneasy. Whether it was his personality or his manner of forcing her into an immediate decision, she came away with a decidedly negative reaction.

Once home, she contacted Sarah Bolieu at the Shriner's Hospital. Here was help she knew she could trust. Sarah was in charge of public relations and many times previously Darla had poured out concerns to her, and was always made to feel better.

Sarah shared information about a research paper that was recently published in England. Its basic premise was that women with abdominal scars from burns were indeed able to carry full term and deliver normally. Any women in the study that had problems was not due to the burns.

Somehow, the study brought out, hormones during pregnancy allow the abdominal scars to give and stretch to make room for the growing child.

All the years of worry had been needless! This study proved it!

She had to let Derek know at once. After a few moments of thanking God for the good news, she went outside to share her happiness with him. She found him outside in the yard, adjusting wheel weights on the tractor.

"I have something wonderful to tell you!" she beamed. "So wonderful! Oh, Derek, He sends one blessing after another, doesn't He?"

But when they decided that now was the time to start a family, each month became another disappointment. It was well into their third year of marriage, and still no sign that a baby had been conceived. In her heart, Darla began to think that it was not God's will that she become a mother.

Dr. Burkhart, an Atlantic physician began a series of tests to find out why there had been no conception. He soon discovered that there was a failure to ovulate. Darla was started on small doses a fertility drug. And she became pregnant.

Although the first months went along without incidence, Dr. Burkhart referred her to a high risk obstetrician in Omaha, Dr. Marvin Dietrich. Her major care came from the Atlantic doctor, with periodic check-ups in the city.

High blood pressure was discovered and the doctor ordered her to work only six hours a day, later reducing it to only four. The Salem Home was cooperative and there was no problem concerning her keeping her job.

With only a month to wait, and excitement mounting, Darla was preparing a room for the baby, and making lists about what to take to the hospital for herself when the Big Day came. An X-ray at this time showed that the baby was lying in a breech position. This, added to Darla's toxemia, signaled the end of her working outside the home.

Limited activity and periodic urine tests were ordered. Dr. Dietrich would see her again the following Monday to perform a non-stress test and yet another ultrasound.

For weeks the family band AcerVale (now Family Tradition) had been scheduled to perform on Saturday afternoon at Orient, Iowa for their annual Pumpkin Days.

"Pumpkin Days!" the doctor exclaimed. "Darla, these are Baby Days!"

With the Hansen philosophy that the show _does_ go on, the engagement was fulfilled. Mardell and Roger drove their motor home to Orient so that Darla could ride in comfort, continue with the urine tests and have a place to lie down between performances.

During the show, she perched rather precariously on a high stool, but the position of the baby made breath control difficult.

CHAPTER 22
MOTHERHOOD

On Monday, with a suitcase along "just in case", Derek drove her to Omaha. The non-stress test, as feared, showed that the baby was in difficulty. The ultrasound also showed there were other problems and they were sent to Methodist Hospital for a pelvic X-ray.

The shocking news was that it appeared there was some sort of tumor or other growth on the baby's neck. Darla was admitted at once to the high risk obstetrics area.

Complete bed rest was the order, with a fetal monitor brought in. An amniocentesis was performed to see if the baby's lungs were mature enough for immediate delivery. Luckily, they were and a C-section was scheduled for the next day, July twenty-third, four weeks ahead of the due date.

Dr. Dietrich came for one last look before going home. "It's going to be a <u>little</u> fellow--or a little miss!" he predicted, peering at her through his glasses. "We're going to have a neonatal pediatrician right in the delivery room to take over on the baby. . ."

His expression told her what he could not bring himself to put into words. The baby was at risk.

They did not have to face the wait alone. Both sets of prospective grandparents, Charles Hansens and

Darla's folks, were there as well as Derek's brother, Tom, and Connie and Ken, Darla's sister and brother.

The support was in sad contrast to Darla's roommate's situation. Unwed, her only help at this most important of times was her father. Darla thanked God for all the people who cared in her life.

Derek was allowed to scrub and don surgical garb so that he might be right there with Darla in the delivery room. She was denied one thing: "Even though you're a nurse, Darla, it would be too hard on you to actually watch the incision." A screen was put in front of her head to block the view.

But Derek could see the whole mysterious, exciting process of a new little life being lifted into the world.

"It's a little girl!" Dr. Dietrich announced.

"Is it really?" Darla asked, tears of happiness coming now. "Is she O.K.?" By that time the pediatrician had hurried her over to the warmer.

"What does she weigh?" Derek's voice was muffled through the mask.

"Right at six pounds, I'd say," the pediatrician answered. And when they did weigh her she was exactly that. She was checked over carefully and all was fine. No tumor, no flaws. A perfect little girl.

Derek was allowed to walk out with the nurse, carrying his first child, to show her to the waiting relatives. "It's a girl! Meet Monica Layne," he introduced her.

Back in her room, Darla lay in a happy, if sleepy state. Of all the problems she had had during the wait, none had been related to her burns.

A year and a half later, a perfect baby boy, Jordan Derek, was delivered vaginally, weighing six pound, twelve ounces. Darla had no problems this time, and worked "to the last minute."

Recently Darla found for the first time what her parents had gone through so many years. For one week, she sat at Monica's bedside, as she recovered from kidney surgery. She was in a great deal of pain, and as Darla sat with her, and as a nurse, assisted in her care, she thought constantly of what her parents must have endured.

Both parents had said, "I would have suffered for you, if I could have, rather than see you go through so much."

Now at last she understood. She could realize what relief and joy was theirs as she made each small triumph towards recovery. Very quickly, Monica bounced back and was once again her energetic and happy self.

CHAPTER 23
MUSIC, MUSIC

For years, Darla sang whenever she got the chance. She sang solos at church, for weddings, and once for a funeral--for a sixteen-year-old girl who died as the result of a car wreck.

She became interested in country music. An Omaha radio station sponsored a contest, and she sent in a demonstration tape, with a friend helping on the piano. The tape won her a place in the contest, with the station providing a back-up band.

An elegant supper club was the site of the contest. She felt hopelessly outclassed, especially when she heard one female entrant had flown in from Nashville to take part.

Although she was not picked as one of the two to advance, this opportunity whetted an appetite for performing in front of an audience.

As she sang "Fly into Love" and "Silver Threads and Golden Needles", she felt excitement and a rapport with the crowd.

God had blessed her with a voice. Was it part of His will for her to use it for public entertainment?

During the time that she was working in Anita, she and another nurse began spending time together after work, making music. The other girl was an excellent pianist, specializing in honky-tonk, which she played by ear.

The two would sing together, having a great time after eight hours of floor duty. Both were interested in getting a band started with other members of Darla's family.

Because Ken was turned off by the strictly country flavor of the piano player's style, the decision was made to form a family group. The nucleus was the trio of Judy, Darla, and Ken. Word got around that they had formed, and were asked to be the entertainment at the Better Elk Horn Club Christmas banquet. They sang a dozen songs, with the emphasis on holiday music, and they were launched!

Connie's husband, Paul Steen, then joined as drummer and arranged for a Valentine's evening performance at an area restaurant. The remuneration was very small, but this second performance gave their reputation a boost.

Excitement grew, with Darla starting to play electric keyboard. Jerry and another nurse friend, Nancy Osborn, joined with guitars. The original name, AcerVale, changed recently to Family Tradition.

In the fall of 1988 Darla added another activity to her busy schedule, teaching a senior citizen exercise class. She did all the choreographing. She studied for and passed a national aerobics certification test from the International Dance and Exercise Association. The seniors do stretch and tone movements to the beat of Big Band and country music. Through the class she was able to provide them with their exercise, but she also gained many fast friendships with some of the participants.

The following summer she added teaching of water aerobics at the Elk Horn pool with her cousin's wife, Emily Hoegh, and aerobics at Walnut and Elk Horn.

The scars that Darla had been left with had made her open to the hurts of others. They had also given her a drive to excel in areas that have nothing to do with the condition of one's epidermis.

Leading her water aerobics class, she dresses in a modern swimsuit, making no attempt to hide her scars.

"If I act natural about it, and don't make a big deal of it, no one else will, either." She is now too busy with family, nursing, and music to worry about what others might think about the texture of her skin.

Young parents in the community began using Darla as an example for not playing with matches. "Look what happened to Darla Hansen!" they would warn children, who showed a fascination for fire.

Darla did not mind being pointed out in this manner. If it could save another child, she could easily be the solemn reminder. She often spoke with them about it herself. So often, people look and stare in wonder about what happened to Darla's skin. Darla says that it is much better if people will ask about it rather than to tell children to "hush" and walk by hurriedly. Darla takes the time to explain questions asked of her.

CHAPTER 24
CHOICES

In addition to their work in the band, Darla and Nancy formed a duo, Girls Nite Out.

When they won over eleven other entrants in a contest in June of 1989, they were ecstatic. They were up against very strong competition and many of the contestants had had a great deal more public exposure than had they.

Family and friends were proud of the pair and predicted that they were now on their way to more and more "number one's" in competition.

Several of their friends from the Salem Home, Myrtue Memorial Hospital, and seventeen senior citizens from the aerobic class drove to Omaha for the next contest. They were there to cheer, to encourage and to share in the thrill of hearing that Girls Nite Out would advance to the contest finals at the Waterloo, Nebraska, fairgrounds in July.

Then came a "shocker." A member of the backup band with which they performed that night, approached the pair with an offer.

"This isn't something I do often," he began. "In fact I've probably only done this twice before in my thirty-odd years of performing. But I'd like to have you with us on our tour through the Midwest this fall." He named the salary that made them momentarily speechless.

"The fact is," he continued, "I'm so sure that you'll add a new, positive dimension to the group that I'm willing to bring the entire band to Elk Horn to practice. But I'll have to have your answer in ten days."

Nancy and her husband, Mitch, who is a high school vocational agriculture instructor and coach, have two pre-school boys. The Hansens' children are also pre-schoolers.

"Why did he have to give us the choice?" Nancy moaned.

"It just wouldn't work, would it?" Darla replied, as much to herself as to Nancy.

But it was tempting. And they approached it from every possible angle -- on the phone, at each of their homes, and with their husbands. It was fun "kicking it around." But neither of them wanted to leave their husband and children to be away for days at a time. The attractive pay checks, however, made them at least speculate what a boost it would give their respective budgets.

"We may never get a chance like this again!"

"Well, when we're old ladies, we can at least remember that we were asked!"

They sat at Nancy's kitchen table, sipping soft drinks and watching the four kids at play.

Neither was really seriously considering the offer. Both put husband and children first on their list of priorities. Yet the offer was gratifying. It reinforced their faith in the music they could make together.

All of the excitement of a road tour, the applause, the chance to meet agents who might offer them an even more lucrative job -- none of it could match what they had at home.

The answer would definitely be "Thanks, but no thanks!" But, oh, it <u>was</u> fun to have been asked!

The girls were later invited to record at Rene Studio in David City, Nebraska. They recorded original music that the two had written as well as some familiar songs. They became more known in the area and continued to perform for banquets and community events. As a duo their voices and friendships mixed well.

CHAPTER 25

ON THE MOUNTAINTOP

Taped back-up music throbbed out over the sound system, giving and intro that set feet tapping and hands clapping in rhythm. Here to watch an undefeated boys' team play a return match against Tri-Center, the crowd was up-beat, happy, a little wild.

Basketball -- both boys and girls -- is so much a part of the life of Elk Horn-Kimballton that in order to seat everyone crowded into the gym, the old custom of the high school band playing before the game and at half time had been dispensed with two years previously -- to the dismay of many band enthusiasts.

Mitch Osborn, boys coach and athletic director and Rod Hoegh, girls coach, principal and also Darla's cousin, now followed the trend at other schools, and substituted soloists for the band music. This night, as many other nights, they had asked Darla to sing "The Star Spangled Banner."

As a prank, Darla and Nancy decided to surprise the crowd by doing a six-song gig while the boys were warming up.

Their voices blended and complemented each other as they belted out one song after another -- including one that Darla herself had written.

Later, one of the team members had told Nancy, "You guys sound great! It was like being at a concert!"

Going to her car after the game, working her way through the crowd, virtually everyone Darla passed had a compliment for her.

"Way to go!"

"Did you write that second song?"

"You two sound professional!"

Finally in her car, Darla sat for a few minutes as the other autos flashed on headlights and eased out of the parking lot.

It had been over twenty-three years since the accident. Would I, she thought, have reacted differently if I had been fourteen, instead of four? Would I have gone into music, become a nurse, married, had children? Or would I have retreated into depression?

Or--the ever-present thought--what if there had been no fire? Would things have been any more wonderful? Or would I have just coasted along, not achieving as I have done?

Darla smiled as she drove along the blacktop road toward home. She knew that no one of us can ever be shown the alternatives. No one ever knows what would have happened, what would have opened, or closed for us, if a certain dramatic moment had not been a part of our lives.

She remembered now an earlier episode that she had shoved to the back of her mind. Her reaction to it had showed not only the others involved, but Darla herself how much importance her scars had for her.

It had been at a gospel concert in Omaha. She had given her Christian testimony and sung a solo.

Afterwards, in the rest room changing clothes before the pot luck supper, she had been cornered by two women from the audience.

According to them, they had <u>both</u> had a vision during Darla's number that she would miraculously be given new skin and her scars would disappear.

"If you have enough faith and pray in the right way, you <u>will</u> be healed!" They announced it, triumphantly.

Darla was stunned.

"I appreciate your concern," she said. "But I <u>have</u> been healed. I was not expected to <u>live</u>! It was a miracle that I survived and am here today!"

The two women were visibly disappointed.

"Don't get me wrong," she continued, as kindly as she could. "I have absolutely no doubts that God could give me new skin, because the Holy Spirit is a healer. But to expect it. . ." She gathered up her case and extra shoes and headed for the door.

Before going out she turned. "Besides," she said, her eyes dancing with a bit of mischief, "I don't think my scars are that bad!"

Wordlessly, the two watched her walk out, head high, and a spring in her step.

Now, driving home, following the tail lights of another carload of fans ahead of her, it seemed as though her thoughts would not shut off. She tried thinking of the game, but her mind kept returning to where she was and how far and hard had been the journey.

Who knows, she mused, what a lazy, dull person I might have been without the fire, without the matches?

She pulled into her yard. Through the window she could see Derek in front of the television, his long legs stretched out in front of him. Upstairs, she knew, the two children would be sleeping soundly, snug and well.

Out of the car, she felt the wind. It whipped around the barn, bending the trees. She pulled her coat more snugly about her, not ready yet to go into the house.

She looked up at the splash of stars flung across the dark February sky. Thousands upon thousands of them, all set in their appointed places, twinkling down at her.

"He made you to do your thing, and me to do mine," she whispered to them.

Then, before going in, still looking up--always looking up--

"Thank you, dear Jesus, for everything. For everything in my life. No exceptions. You've been so good to me, Lord!"

With one slender hand, she lightly touched the scars on her neck, as if to remind herself that they were still there, would always be there.

"Yes, in everything, Lord, I say thank you!" In the silence, in the darkness, she knew He heard.

She turned to go into the house, full of joy.

THE
END